Preface

"WE'RE ALL GONNA die!" is just the sort of thing that a typical, hopeless bystander would utter in a movie about the post-apocalypse, before getting his head chewed off by a computer-generated monster. It's just the sort of line written by countless overworked screenwriters, mired in some sort of authenticity, giving the audience a sense of true hopelessness in a battered world. However, this line is more than just an off-the-hip outburst by an on-screen character. It gives the viewer a strange malaise. Nobody I know would say such a thing, one would think, *it's just a line in a movie*. However, our hypothetical screenwriter might have much more wisdom than we give them credit for.

Countless forms of the pandemic story have played out through every conceivable form of media, from movies to television shows and countless novels. Examples of such pandemics include Ebola and the Bird Flu, to the oft-forgotten Spanish flu of 1918. But the stories never stop there. Like twisted playthings, screenwriters love to exaggerate the nature and properties of these pandemics to dizzying new heights, like the quintessential zombie apocalypse scenario. These stories have also been explored in virtual and interactive spaces, like my son's favorite game series Resident Evil, where the ambitious and flawed experiments of evil corporations result in lab-grown viral pandemics that wreak havoc throughout the world. There is seemingly no end to the madness.

Although fiction writers have their own affinity with *this* exaggerated pandemic, there is a split between the more pragmatic medical vernacular of the scientific community, and the party-line dialectic of the political sphere. Everyone wants a piece of the action, especially in modern times, where pandemic language has become as commonplace as asking about the weather.

It is in this paradoxical world, most people forget about the Spanish Flu. Of course, scientists are there to remind us of how catastrophic the death toll was of that not-so-distant event in history, but who's to listen, especially when armed with one's own version of the truth! With a death toll that surpassed that of World War I, humanity should be more apt to pay attention to that stark nearly one-hundred-year-old lesson.

Despite those catastrophic numbers, we revert into a state of stark denial, like that hapless viewer eating up that post-apocalyptic movie. *That could never happen to us*, we think, as we have another handful of popcorn. *Surely, the world could never lose another fifty-million people from a single pandemic ever again*. Of course, the world is a different place today, as we have made multiple groundbreaking

The New Pandemic

Concise Review of Viral, Bacterial and Parasitic Infections

Endemics

Epidemics

Epidemiology & Pandemics

COVID-19

Asif Anwar, MD

outskirts press

The New Pandemic
Concise Review of Viral, Bacterial and Parasitic Infections.
Endemics - Epidemics - Epidemiology & Pandemics COVID-19
All Rights Reserved.
Copyright © 2022 Asif Anwar, MD
v2.0

The opinions expressed in this manuscript are solely the opinions of the author and do not represent the opinions or thoughts of the publisher. The author has represented and warranted full ownership and/or legal right to publish all the materials in this book.

This book may not be reproduced, transmitted, or stored in whole or in part by any means, including graphic, electronic, or mechanical without the express written consent of the publisher except in the case of brief quotations embodied in critical articles and reviews.

Outskirts Press, Inc.
http://www.outskirtspress.com

Paperback ISBN: 978-1-9772-4216-7
Hardback ISBN: 978-1-9772-4237-2

Cover Photo © 2022 www.gettyimages.com. All rights reserved - used with permission.

Outskirts Press and the "OP" logo are trademarks belonging to Outskirts Press, Inc.

PRINTED IN THE UNITED STATES OF AMERICA

medical discoveries since the turn of the 20th century, like antibiotics, symptomatic treatment options and other drastic, yet innovative procedures. In fact, we have done such a good job, that our population grows larger and older, as we head into the new "roaring" twenties.

But how quickly does humanity forget an event like the Spanish Flu? The most recent major viral outbreak (SARS) serves as our answer. Instead of SARS being one of many headstones in the annals of our medical history, it should instead have served as humanity's wake-up call. Granted, SARS did not have a major effect on most people's lives in the western world, with virtually no bottleneck to our healthcare or economic systems. We humans were quick to assume their imperviousness. However, SARS served as the perfect template of what could go wrong in an ever-changing new world.

This brings us to the novel coronavirus, or COVID-19. Even when there were distant calls on the horizon of an outbreak in the Wuhan Province in China, the media and our politicians morphed into that proverbial movie-goer from before. Information fell into the mire of party-lines and selective science. As a result, few of us took note. By us, I mean the healthcare system at large, federal and state governments with disaster and infrastructural plans, school principals, CEO's and ironically, movie studios in Hollywood. We all succumbed to that ostrich mentality, that deadly psychological snag called groupthink. We all turned into a theatre full of casual moviegoers, all watching the same CNN or FOX, depending on our political inclination, clips reporting of disaster at Wuhan, as we shoved more chocolate-covered raisins into our eager mouths.

While this is not a psychology book. We must take note of the herd immunity concept. Well, not *that* herd immunity, but our aforementioned concept of groupthink, where we collectively believe that we are somehow immune to whatever catastrophe is spreading around in the world. Even when the virus infiltrated into neighboring Asian countries like Iran, and even into Europe, like the deadly outbreak in Italy, Americans chose to avoid the lessons until the disease was knocking on New York's shores. Only when the dead piled higher, did we come to the harsh realization that we were not prepared for this new pandemic. This was not just another Severe Acute Respiratory Syndrome (SARS) or Middle Eastern Respiratory Syndrome (MERS) or, much to the ire of many, just another form of the seasonal flu.

Even when COVID persisted and came to the US, the media and our politicians labelled it a disease targeting the elderly, that only people in nursing homes or those with underlying comorbid conditions should take precautions. We are quickly learning that all this speculation proved wrong when COVID started to infect relatively young and healthy individuals once thought safe. Whether you like him or not, President Trump rightfully touted COVID as the new war, with an enemy invisible to the naked eye. Whether he treated it as one, is another story entirely.

The world could have never anticipated such a deadly and mysterious disease, even though we could have, if that makes sense. So, as our economy tumbled and our healthcare systems were tested, more and more of us wished that we heeded more lessons from the past.

COVID dismantled our society exactly in the same way it functions in the human body. The virus causes the human body to unleash "storms" of cytokines, transforming human immune-response systems into lethal weapons. Essentially, it uses what's originally inside of the human body to propagate itself and kill the host as a byproduct. Similarly, COVID unleashed a surge of cytokine storms into our society, revealing those vulnerabilities in infrastructure and the lack of emergency preparedness that have always existed. Unlike the war it's being touted as, this outbreak shares little with conventional or asymmetrical warfare. COVID does not present a linear battle. There is no back and forth, no preparation. We have seen warfare in every form all across the globe. The American Military is the most sophisticated and prepared force the world has ever seen. But the analogy falls apart in the end. We cannot challenge a microscopic enemy by treating it like an insurgency, or an abnormality. This enemy turns our own bodies against us. It is poetic really, in a changing society, our rules of economics and finance and even ordering groceries has changed, so it is only fitting that we have a virus that changes all the rules. Hopefully our "fight" against COVID will serve as our Battle of Stalingrad rather than our Waterloo.

The societal components of the pandemic have a confluence effect even though it can originate in varied cultures and geographical locations. Albeit the one common denominator across the board is human suffering and grave societal impact, which exposes its strengths and weaknesses, whether that is dead bodies sitting in the freezers outside New York hospitals or floating swollen corpses in the Ganges.

The purpose of writing this is to put my observations into some sort of historical and scientific perspective. Also, to enhance understanding of the basic concepts of pandemics and infections, with an opportunity to expand on these issues in the future. My hope is to present a clear set of medical definitions untainted by the media, various organizations, or politicians, so anyone reading this book can know when to put the popcorn down and realize the CGI monster can be the real thing.

-Asif Anwar

Dedication
To my parents, Major (R) Anwar
&
Kalsum Anwar

Disclaimer

THIS PUBLICATION IS intended to be educational in nature and is not a substitute for clinical decision making based on the medical condition presented. It is the responsibility of the user/reader to ensure all information contained herein is current and accurate by using published references. Manufacturers' documentation and drug information provided by pharmaceutical companies should be referenced prior to using any equipment or medication. Due to the ever-changing field of medicine, some of the treatment modalities may change or be altered by CDC-FDA and other regulatory agencies. It is suggested and recommended to review late information before any treatment regimen is initiated. Therefore, authors and publishers bear no responsibility for any potential harm rendered due to any content in this book

Authors and Contributors

Asif Anwar, MD, MS, FCCP, FCCM, CPE
Lt Col-Senior Flight Surgeon-Critical Care Air Transport
128 ARW Milwaukee WI, ANG-USAF
Department Chief-Pulmonary and Sleep Medicine
Program Director-Pulmonary Fellowship
Captain James A. Lovell FHCC-VA, Medical Center North Chicago, IL
Assistant Professor of Medicine-Chicago Medical School-Rosalind Franklin University
Consultant-Attending Pulmonary, Critical Care and Sleep Medicine
Vista Medical Center-Waukegan IL
Condell Medical Center-Advocate-Aurora-Libertyville IL

Sherezaad A. Anwar, JD,
Editor-in-Chief Transnational Law & Contemporary Problems
The Iowa University-School of Law
Iowa City, Iowa

Azib Shahid, MD
Internal Medicine Resident
Rosalind Franklin University/Chicago Medical School, IL
Captain James A. Lovell FHCC-VA, Medical Center North Chicago, IL

Madeeha Banu, MD
Internal Medicine Resident
Rosalind Franklin University/Chicago Medical School, IL
Captain James A. Lovell FHCC-VA, Medical Center North Chicago, IL

Emmanuel N. Njoku, MD,
Attending Physician-Infectious Diseases
Assistant Professor of Medicine-Chicago Medical School-Rosalind Franklin University
Captain James A. Lovell FHCC-VA-Medical Center North Chicago, IL

Haili Campanella, MSN-FNP, BSN-RN, CCRN
Nurse Practitioner Pulmonary, Critical Care and Sleep Medicine
Vista Medical Center-Waukegan IL

Catherine M. Goodale MSN-Acute Care NP
Nurse Practitioner Pulmonary Critical Care
Vista Medical Center-Waukegan IL

Ralph Seymoure, PA
Physician Assistant - Pulmonary, Critical Care, Sleep Medicine and ER
Vista Medical Center-Waukegan IL

Khalida A. Anwar, MD, MS
Consultant Physician
Physical Medicine & Rehabilitation
Pain Management

Eishaa Sajjad
Pre-Med Student
COMSATS University

Zoha Hassan
Undergraduate Student
Loyola University, Chicago IL

Reviewers

Jack C. O'horo MD, MPH, FACP
Consultant, Division of Infectious Diseases
Joint Appointment in Pulmonary and Critical Care Medicine
Associate Professor of Medicine, Mayo Clinic College of Medicine

Col. Michael Borkowski, MD
Wisconsin State Air Surgeon
Senior Flight Surgeon
128 Air Refueling Wing
Air National Guard USAF-Milwaukee WI

Acknowledgements

Lavanya Srinavasan, MD
Assistant Professor of Medicine -Chicago Medical School-Rosalind Franklin University
Consultant-Attending Pulmonary, Critical Care and Sleep Medicine
Vista Medical Center-Waukegan IL
Condell Medical Center-Advocate-Aurora-Libertyville IL

Srikanth Davuluri, MD
Assistant Professor of Medicine-Chicago Medical School-Rosalind Franklin University
Consultant-Attending Pulmonary, Critical Care and Sleep Medicine
Vista Medical Center-Waukegan IL
Condell Medical Center-Advocate-Aurora-Libertyville IL

Kunal Patel, MD
Assistant Professor of Medicine-Chicago Medical School-Rosalind Franklin University
Consultant-Attending Pulmonary, Critical Care and Sleep Medicine
Vista Medical Center-Waukegan IL
Condell Medical Center-Advocate-Aurora-Libertyville IL

Michael Ries, MD, MBA, FCCM, FCCP, FACP
Medical Director, System Critical Care
Tele-Critical Care, Patient Command Center
Advocate-Aurora Health System, Oak Brook IL

Aristides Assimacopoulas, MD
Infectious Disease Specialist
Metro Infectious Disease Consultants, L.L.C
Chicago, IL

Mirza Qasim Hasan, MD, MPH, FACP
Assistant Professor of Medicine
Program Director - Apogee Physicians
University of Texas Health Sciences Center at Houston

Raul Gazmuri, MD, PhD, FCCM,
Section Chief-Critical Care & Director ICU
Professor of Medicine-Chicago Medical School-Rosalind Franklin University
Captain James A. Lovell FHCC-VA- Medical Center North Chicago, IL

Rodney D. Boyum MD, PhD
Attending Physician-Pathology
Professor of Medicine-Chicago Medical School-Rosalind Franklin University Captain James A. Lovell FHCC-VA-Medical Center North Chicago, IL

Editing - Proofreading - Design - Cover

Liz Osborn
e-ICU
Advocate Intensive Partners
Advocate Aurora Health-Oakbrook IL

Wasif Anwar, BS-Engineering
Architectural-Electric Engineer
Hartford- CT

Hina Anwar, MFA, MPhil, PhD (S)
Anthropologist-Museum Lok Virsa

Vicki Lavi
Author of "Searching for Virginia"
Vista Memorial Hospital
Waukegan Illinois

Present and Past Affiliations-Academia-Medical Institutions

Captain James A. Lovell-FHCC.
VA North Chicago-IL
Rosalind Franklin University-Chicago Medical School
North Chicago, IL

Vista Medical Center
Waukegan, IL

Advocate-Aurora Health- eICU
Oakbrook, IL
Good Shepherd Hospital-Barrington IL
Lutheran General Hospital- Park Ridge IL
St. Luke's Hospital-Milwaukee WI

Baptist Medical Center-Nassau
Fernandina Beach-Florida

United Hospital-Froedtert South (St Catherine's-Kenosha Medical)
Kenosha-Pleasant Prairie WI

Northwestern University
Evanston, IL

Northeastern IL. University
Chicago, IL

Saint Louis University
Saint Louis-Missouri
Forest Park Hospital

Morristown Memorial Hospital
Morristown, NJ

UMDNJ-University of Medicine & Dentistry
Brunswick, New Jersey

Sind Medical College-UK
Karachi-PK

Military College Jhelum
Sarai-Alamagir-PK

Scott's Air Force Base
Illinois

934 Airlift Wing
Minneapolis - Minnesota

128 Air Refueling Wing
Milwaukee - Wisconsin

115 Fighter Wing
Jacksonville - Florida

Contents

Preface i
Disclaimer ix
Authors And Contributors xi
Reviewers xiv
Acknowledgements xv

PART I 1
The Basics -Definitions - Terminology 1
   Microbiology 1
   Virus 2
   Virology 2
   Bacteria 3
   Fungi 4
   Mycology 4
   Protozoa 5
   Helminths 5
   Amoeba 6
   Parasites 7
      Endo-Parasites 7
      Ecto-Parasite 7
   Prion 7
   Viral Load-(VL) 8
   Viral Inoculum 8
   Virulence 9

    Infectivity..9
    Pathogenicity 9
    Carriers of disease - vector.............................10
    Spectrum of disease 11
    Antigen..11
    Antibody 11
    Toxins..12
    Spores 13

Medications or Drug Approval Process 15
    Emergency Use Authorization (EUA)................15
    Experimental Use Authorization (EUA) 16
    Investigational New Drug (IND).........................16
    Empiric Treatment...16
    Prophylaxis Treatment 17
        Pre-exposure...17
        Post-exposure 17
    Definitive Treatment...18
    Concordant Treatment 18
    Discordant Treatment..18

Epidemiology & Statistics 19
    Clinical Studies 19
    Anecdotes, Editorials, Ideas, Opinions (AEIO) ...21
    Case Reports and Case Series 21
    Cross-Sectional Studies.....................................22
    Case-Control Studies 22
    Cohort Studies (Prospective and Retrospective)..22
    Confounding Variable 23

Blinding in clinical research studies..................24
      Single blind, double blind...........................24
  Allocation Concealment.....................................24
  Randomized Control Trials 24
  Meta-Analysis-Review Studies 25
  Retrospective Studies..25
  Prospective Studies...25
  Null Hypothesis...26
  Correlation Study..26
  Type I Error...26
  Type II Error..27

Types of Biases in the research studies and analytics 28
  Selection Bias...28
  Confirmation Bias...28
  Outliers 29
  Overfitting and Underfitting Bias 29
  Confounding Bias...29

Statistical Terminology 30
  p-Value..30
  Incidence 30
  Prevalence..30
  Sensitivity aka PID (Positive in Disease) 30
  Specificity aka NIH (Negative In Health)..........31
  Positive Predictive Value - PPV.........................31
  Negative Predictive Value - NPV......................31
  Relative Risk Reduction - RRR 31

    Absolute Risk Reduction - ARR 32
    Numbers to Needed to Treat - NTT 32
    Numbers to Harm - NNH 32
    Confidence Interval - CI 32
    A-Accurate *aka Precise aka Bullseye* 33
    B-Precision *aka Reliability* 33
    C-Accuracy *aka Validity* 33
    D-Neither Accurate nor Precise *aka Not Valid-Not Reliable* 34

Statistical Tests - commonly and frequently used .. 34
    Chi-square 34
    Student t-test 34
    Mann-Whitney U test - Wilcoxon Test 34
    Statistical Presentation of data 35
    Kaplan Meier Curve 35
    Pie chart or pie graph 36
    Bar vs Line Graph 36
    Scatter plot 37

Types of Statistical Data 38
    Linear 38
    Non-Linear Data 38

Epidemic Terminology 38
    Index Case 38
    Mortality Rate 38
    Case Fatality Ratio 39
    Incidence 39

Prevalence 39
Apex 39
Asymptomatic Carrier State 39
Community Spread 40
Epidemic aka "Outbreak" 40

Epidemic Patterns.. 40
Point Source Epidemic 40
Common Source Epidemic 41
Progressive or Propagational Epidemics 41
Mixed Epidemics 41

Source-Contact Tracing 41
Antigenic Variation.. 41
Antigenic Drift 41
Antigenic Shift 42
Pandemic Shifts... 43
Pandemic Resurgence-Recurrence 43
Antigenic Divergence... 44
Antigenic Stasis.. 44
Antigenic Evolution.. 45
Genetic Viral Diversity 45
Genetic and Racial Diversity.................................. 45
Gain of Function 46
Endemic illness.. 46
Pandemic disease 47
Epicenter 47
Person Under Investigation - PUI 47
Confirmed Case.. 48

- Harm Reduction 48
- Vectors 48
- Biological Host 49
  - Accidental 49
  - Incidental 49
  - Reservoir 49
  - Primary 49
  - Host Factors 49

Zoonotic Spillover and Transmissibility 49
Biological Warfare-Bioterrorism 50
Diagnosing an Epidemic 51
Critical Supplies 52
Personal Protective Equipment (PPE) 53
- Masks 53
- Respirators 55
- Ventilators 55
- Universal Precautions 55

Triage Decisions 56
Herd Immunity - Community Immunity 58
Immune-compromised Host (ICH) 59
Hygiene Hypothesis 60
Germ Theory of Disease 60
Epidemics and Societal Impact 61
Population and Disease 61
Fear Factor - Fear of Unknown 61
Treatment Modalities 63
Vaccines 63

Antibody Treatment 67
Convalescent Plasma 68
Genomic Surveillance 68
Anti Vaxxers-Vaccine Hesitancy 68
Public Health Policy vs Public Relations Postures 70
Psychological Impact 71
Biological Warfare 71
Medical Impact - COVID Hospital Hesitancy 71
Social Determinants of Health 72
Economic Implications 73
Mitigation Strategies 74
Shelter In Place-Stay Home-Lock down 74
Isolation Impact 75
Social Distancing 75
Spiritual Connection 76
Geographical Templating 76
Population Health 77
Policy vs Politics 77
Military Engagement 78
Quarantine 78
Self-Quarantine 78
Obligatory Quarantine 79
Behavioral Modification 79
Flattening the Curve 80
Measures taken during an epidemics 81
Conspiracy Theories 82
Telemedicine or Telehealth 83
Tele-education 84

**Regulatory Agencies-Governmental
   Organizations-NGO**..85
   State and County Regulated Agencies 85
   FDA - Food and Drug Administration...............86
   HHS - Health and Human Services...................86
   CDC - Center for Disease Control.....................86
   FEMA - Federal Emergency Management
      Agency 87
   OSHA - Occupational Safety Health
      Administration 87
   NFPA - National Fire Protection Association 88
   JC - JOINT COMMISSION 88

Zoonotic Disease 89

PART II..94
Coronavirus *aka Covid-19 - SARS-CoV-2* 94
Spanish Flu-1918..153
Asian Flu (1956-1958)...158
Flu Pandemic (1968) 161
Avian Flu 164
SARS-CoV 167
MERS..170
Lassa Fever..173
Ebola Virus 177
Hantavirus 183
Yellow Fever..188
AIDS 191
Zika Virus..196

- Dengue Fever 199
- Chikungunya Virus 203
- Malaria 206
- West Nile Disease 211
- Eastern Equine Encephalitis 215
- Anthrax 218
- Plague 224
- Smallpox 231
- Monkeypox 234
- Chicken Pox 237
- Polio - Poliomyelitis 242
- Measles 248
- Mumps 252
- Rubella 255
- Typhoid & Paratyphoid Fever 258
- Norwalk Virus 262
- Tuberculosis - TB 265
- Syphilis 270
- Rabies 275
- Hepatitis A Virus (Hep-A) 279
- Hepatitis B Virus (HBV) 283
- Hepatitis C Virus (HBC) 288
- Hepatitis D Virus 293
- Hepatitis E Virus 297
- Clostridium Difficile 301
- Clostridium Tetani 305
- Clostridium Botulism 308
- Clostridium Perfringens 311
- Enterohemorrhagic Fever 315

Marburg Virus 319
Cholera 323
Legionnaires Disease 328
Prion Diseases.. 332
Trypanosomiasis... 338
American Trypanosomiasis 344
Lyme Disease 348
Primary Amoebic Meningoencephalitis............... 353
Leishmaniasis... 357

Abbreviations... 362
References 366

PART I

The Basics - Definitions - Terminology

THE FIRST SECTION of this publication contains definitions of common medical and public health terms, which are often used without proper meaning by news media outlets and political pundits.

Microbiology

The study of microbes or organisms which are only visible under a microscope, i.e., bacteria, fungi, viruses, and parasites, is called microbiology. Microbiologists work to identify the organisms responsible for disease and study their properties and weaknesses to guide current and future therapies. Microbiologists also evaluate these organisms for potential benefits, and deleterious effects on the animal and plant kingdoms.

Virus

An agent made up of nucleic acid and a glycoprotein "coat." The simplicity of this organism's structure renders it small enough that it can only be viewed with an electron microscope. But simple is not always good, as the organism's small and simple structure makes it elusive and harmful. Viruses are obligate parasites, meaning that they are required to live inside another organism for survival, as they have none of the organelles or cellular structures of free-living bacteria or eukaryotes. Viruses carry either a code for ribonucleic acid (RNA) or deoxyribonucleic acid (DNA) which hijack the cellular machinery of a host cell to transform it into a replication factory. Viruses also express evasion attributes, making them extremely difficult to control or eradicate. The research center of the Smithsonian Institution recently reported the discovery of several 15,000-year-old viruses from the Tibetan Glacier. According to the report, 28 out of the 33 viruses from that glacier were new to humans. This discovery opens a window to the past as these viruses have been prevalent way before recorded history or modern medicine.

Virology

The branch of science that relates to the study of viruses. Viruses are obligate parasites with *phagocytic* properties. Phagocytosis is a term tied to the eating or consumption of material. The closest analogy would be the good old video game "Pac Man," where the player eats or engulfs everything that comes in its path. Viruses need a definitive host for survival and replication, as they are not capable of surviving on their own. They often use other animals, including pigs, birds, bats and humans to meet their survival needs. Viruses can also use organisms as small as bacteria as hosts. These *bacteriophages* (viruses which can eat bacteria) infect and use bacteria for replication. Viruses consist of an outer protein moiety and an inner nucleic acid which is either single or double stranded, which are called RNA or DNA virus respectively. Viruses have the capability to infect both animals as well as the plant species.

Bacteria

Small unicellular organisms, which are composed of cell walls, cell membranes and nucleic acids. Bacteria are definitely much more complex organisms than viruses. Bacteria are devoid of cellular organelles which are unique to more advanced eukaryotic species i.e., rodents and human beings amongst others. The aggregation of these organelles in advanced species, such as humans, makes it possible for cells to specialize and develop into organs and systems in multicellular life. They can survive in diverse atmospheric conditions and have been found in every biome on earth. The variety of bacteria that have adapted to all sorts of different atmospheric environments means that a staggering number of strains and species exist. Believe it or not, these strains can be used for human benefit in processes like making cheese and yogurt, in addition to the better-known bacterial infections that cause disease.

Fungi

Fungi are organisms with their own class and genera including microbes close to bacterial size, but with more complicated intracellular structures such as cell walls. Some fungi are pathogenic (disease causing) in humans like invasive aspergillosis. Others are critical to maintaining an appropriate balance in the body, like yeasts that help maintain gastrointestinal flora. Yeast is a critical ingredient in baking and cheese making. Diagnosis and treatment of fungal diseases can be very challenging, as the more complex cell structures are closer to human cell structure, and so antifungal agents must be managed carefully to avoid side effects toxic to the patient.

Mycology

The study of fungi, their elements and properties. Out of the 70,000 species of Fungi, 300 are known to cause diseases in humans. Opportunistic fungal diseases pose a threat to healing processes due to the wide use of antibiotics and immunosuppressive agents.

Protozoa
Single celled organisms which either live independently or as a parasite to a host organism. They are ubiquitous to the environment. They thrive on and eat bacteria, fungi and other protozoa. Pathogenic protozoa infect human beings through water and food-borne sources. Like fungi, the more complex cell structures of protozoa make diagnosis and treatment difficult. Most protozoa are toxic to other protozoa and will also be somewhat toxic to human cells, needing careful dosing and monitoring. Protozoa are further classified based on their morphology and structure into amoeba, flagellates and ciliates.

Helminths
Multicellular parasites which are macroscopic and usually recognized as worms, including pinworms, roundworms, tapeworms and flukes. These organisms are responsible for causing various diseases based on certain geographies and host conditions. For example, pinworms and tapeworms are common pathogenic organisms in third world countries. They tend to reside in the intestines of the host. They consume all essential nutrients i.e., iron and proteins, depleting their hosts and resulting in iron deficiency anemia in children. An aggressive initiative by the WHO and UNESCO to treat all school-going children in third world countries with anthelminthic drugs such as Albendazole has reduced the incidence of iron deficiency anemia

in those often malnourished children. In some reports the average school grade child improved significantly after a simple prophylactic/empiric intervention of a once monthly pill or an anthelminthic (antiparasitic) drug.

Amoeba

These unicellular (eukaryote) "blob-like" organisms have the unique ability to alter their shape by the process of extending and retracting pseudopods. Think of a starfish when it moves underwater by extending its arms or tentacles. This unique side-to-side movement is called *diapedesis*. They can also be referred to as *"shape shifters,"* due to their flexibility to contort to any surrounding structure.

Amoebae can also cause diseases in humans. The most common amoeba is called *entamoeba histolytica,* which can cause infection of the human gut and liver, presenting with dysentery. There are other harmless gut amoebae such as *entamoeba dispar* which coexist with their host without causing any problems. Primary Amoebic Meningoencephalitis, *aka Brain-Eating Amoeba,* is one example of a virulent amoeba that causes severe brain disease.

Parasites

Endo-Parasites
These organisms live inside a host organism and cause a variety of diseases. These parasites can be microscopic (only visible under a microscope), like protozoan parasites, or macroscopic (visible with naked eye), like helminths i.e., pinworms or hookworms.

Ecto-Parasite
A parasite that lives outside the body of its host. Typically, the target host belongs to a different species than that of the *ectoparasite*. Examples of these parasites may be fleas, ticks, or body lice. Sometimes this relationship may be symbiotic or mutually beneficial. On the other hand, this relationship can be detrimental, and even fatal. The ectoparasite may not kill its host but rely on its nutrition and use it as a habitat. For example, small remora "attach" to sharks fins and underbellies in order to catch a few scraps of food after the host's feast, or to eat parasites off the shark's skin. Symbiotic indeed!

Prion
These "catch-all" protein moieties cannot be classified as bacteria, viruses, helminth, fungi or protozoa. These are pathogenic agents which can cause abnormalities of cellular protein folding when they reproduce. The most notable side effect that occurs

in human beings is neurodegeneration that occurs in the brain. Human examples include Creutzfeldt-Jakob disease (mad-cow disease), Kuru (cannibalism), Familial Fatal Insomnia, and Gerstmann-Straussler-Scheinker Syndrome. These diseases are always fun to learn about, with deadly and strange symptoms to boot.

Viral Load-(VL)
aka viral titer or viral burden or viral dose

Viral load is a numerical representation of the quantity of a virus measured in a specimen of blood, plasma, sputum, water sample or other kinds of body fluids (fun). It is usually reported as a qualitative measure, such as detectable or undetectable, or as a numeric measurement. For example, the HIV virus is reported as the number of RNA copies per milliliter (ml) of blood. Typically, viral load correlates with how infectious a particular substance is. The higher the number of copies of the virus or viral load, the higher the prediction of the disease and infectivity.

Viral Inoculum

Defined as the *infective dose* of the virus. This merely represents the notion that there exists a sufficient quantity of virus being released from an infected person, animal or environment that can cause a disease in the recipient. For example, there exists a sufficient viral inoculum shed from a SARS-CoV-2 (COVID-19) patient while coughing or sneezing that may render others more susceptible to contracting the disease. The practice of mask wearing by both infected people and potential hosts can prevent spread of the disease by reducing the quantity of the inoculum present in the environment.

Virulence

The innate or inherent ability of a pathogen to infect, harm or kill an organism. In other words, it's the degree of pathogenicity of bacteria, virus, or fungi. Hence, virulence is the degree or the ability of causing a disease. The higher the virulence of the organism, the higher the ability to cause damage to the host. Virulence has made headlines a COVID-19 has mutated around the world. For example, the Delta strain has been reported to have a high level of virulence or infectivity, causing health officials to recommend more stringent practices for the average American.

Infectivity

The ability of a virus to cause infection. Pretty self-explanatory. This term is often used interchangeably with virulence. The CDC describes infectivity as the proportion of exposed persons who become infected.

Pathogenicity

The ability of an infectious agent to cause disease. In practice, having an infection doesn't always mean *disease*. Pathogenicity can be expressed as the portion of affected individuals who develop clinically significant disease. There are many factors in pathogenicity, including the inherent property of the microorganism, or conditions perfect for replication. This includes variety and construction of host immune response and defense mechanisms.

Carriers of disease - vector

A person or animal who gets infected but may or may not exhibit any symptoms or signs of overt disease. Even if the symptoms do occur, they are often subclinical. Carriers have the potential to spread disease more effectively than those who pose symptoms, due to the covert nature of their supposed health. It is often these carriers who can turn an outbreak into a pandemic. These silent, symptomatic spreaders were chief in the proliferation of SARS-CoV-2.

The proverbial 'Typhoid Mary' serves as a great example of this concept. She was the center of major typhoid spread, and a textbook example of an asymptomatic carrier amplifying transmission. Favorite haunts of carriers include major football games, the Lollapalooza music festival and the world's largest religious gathering, the "Kumbh Mela" in India, which may have been responsible for the Delta variant.

Spectrum of disease
Clinical manifestation of disease can present in many ways, ranging from unrecognizable carrier states, to subclinical or overt clinical manifestation. It could be a milder form of the disease or could be severe and critical. The outcome of any disease results in either complete vs impartial recovery, disability or sometimes may even prove to be fatal.

Antigen
A substance, particle, or moiety from a foreign agent like bacteria, virus or fungi which induces and triggers immune responses. Typically, proteins or nucleic acid sequences that are foreign to that organism or animal are recognized by the immune system as such, triggering that overwhelming immune response. If someone is given blood or blood products from an unmatched donor, it can result in an antigenic response in the recipient and result in an antigen-antibody reaction. Same with organ donation. Therefore a lot of energy is spent on seeking compatibility.

Antibody
A protein structure produced by the immune system that binds to antigens as part of the immune response. This phenomenon makes this ligand or the antigen-antibody visible to the innate and acquired immune forces, making it susceptible for destruction. In humans, this is typically mediated by production of IgM

antibodies initially, followed by a stronger and more specific immune response mediated by IgG. Other types of antibodies exist, such as IgA (involved in mucous membrane responses) and IgE (implicated in allergies and disordered immune response) but are typically less consequential to functional immunity. Antibodies can be induced by either infection or vaccination. There is a difference between an antibody being produced by vaccination and infection. In the latter instance, the outcome in the host can be unpredictable. These outcomes can range from a subtle fever or rash to something called an overt immunological mediated catastrophic manifestation or anaphylaxis. This can result in significant morbidity and/or mortality. On the other hand, vaccines produce more controlled or predictable immune responses, with occasional idiosyncratic reactions. Like an adverse reaction to a flu shot, in someone with an egg allergy.

Toxins

Toxins are poisons originating from living or nonliving sources with a unique property to harm other cells and organisms. Toxins can damage directly (i.e., organelle damage) or indirectly (by the production of an antibody-mediated phenomenon). Some toxins are produced by animals as a part of a defense mechanism, such as the poisonous response via snake bite or a fugu "puffer" fish gland. Toxins may also be released when the integrity of the organs or structures

THE BASICS -DEFINITIONS - TERMINOLOGY

harboring these toxins is compromised during necrosis, as happens with inflammation and infection of the abdomen in peritonitis after a ruptured appendix.

Toxicity is a function of both how "poisonous" the molecule is, the duration of exposure and the dose of those toxins given to the organism or the host. Toxic effects can be used productively in medicine, such as in antibiotics which are toxic to bacteria, or the poison dart frog's toxin, *curare*, which can be used as a neuromuscular blocking agent when used as a muscle relaxing agent for an anesthetic. "Any drug can be a poison or toxin and any poison or toxin can be drug/medicine" when cleaved correctly and proportionally.

Spores

These are minute, unicellular particles of bacteria, viruses or fungi which often remain environmentally resistant or dormant for prolonged periods of time, sometimes months and years. This long dormancy is especially present when environmental conditions are not conducive to the spore's growth and proliferation. Once conditions change to become suitable for the growth of the spore, the spore may become desirable or undesirable, depending. The spore reproduces asexually, as compared with gametes which who have to go through their usual rigmarole (sorry humans). There are several examples of spores causing diseases when activated properly within their human hosts. *Histomycosis/histoplasmosis, candidiasis, aspergillosis, and blastomycosis* are some. As stated before, these spores are endemic to certain regions and are quite ubiquitous. They may gain access in humans without causing any disease like Histoplasma, a common presence in the Ohio River Valley. Histoplasma can be found in the respiratory tract of random asymptomatic individuals when sampled. However, multiple factors and conditions must exist before they germinate, flourish, and cause disease.

Exo-spores
Exo-Spores are an outer covering or layer of the spore, a "hard shell" for you chocolate connoisseurs, keeping the biological vanilla ice cream of the spore safe from external damage and degradation.

These detrimental conditions can result from extreme temperatures, humidity, and other detrimental forces of nature.

Endo-spores
Often formed inside an organism, bacteria or fungi when substantive nutrients are depleted. Endo spores are a survival mechanism and an adaptive strategy, which involve complex developmental processes, when the surrounding environment is not conducive for growth and survival. These environmental threats include extreme temperatures, ultraviolet light, enzymatic destruction and chemical degradation.

Medications or Drug Approval Process

Emergency Use Authorization (EUA)
A declaration or authority power bestowed to the FDA (USA) to use a particular medication or test on an emergent basis. The obvious modern day example would be the COVID-19 PCR, an antibody test that was granted emergency use by the CDC. The usual FDA approval process is a well-researched and time-tested process.

The safety and efficacy of any medicine or suggested therapy is evaluated using various research methodologies and statistical tools. However, EUA or Emergency Use Authorization is done double-time if the potential benefits outweigh risks. Examples include the emergency use of HIV medicines during the early period of the disease, when antiretroviral medications were prescribed based on the positive outcomes in two patients. EUA was considered for COVID-19 medication Remdesivir and for the vaccines.

Experimental Use Authorization (EUA)

Another kind of authorization when certain treatment is approved only under emergent circumstances. Experimental use of convalescent plasma is one example of such use in COVID patients. There is a set of stringent guidelines and rules that govern this authorization. A study protocol is often implemented in the conduct of its use.

Investigational New Drug (IND)

IND is a formal application which is submitted to regulatory agencies like the FDA for approval of a specific drug for an investigational use. Among the review process are considered experiences and reports, as well as anecdotal data to support its use. For example, "allogeneic mesenchymal stem cell therapy", i.e., *remestemcel-L* for ARDS in COVID-19 patients.

Empiric Treatment

The word *Empiric* is derived from the Greek word for *experience*. In laymen's terms, this is a treatment regimen based on a series of educated guesses, implemented at the onset of disease symptoms. Medications or antibiotics which are chosen as empiric agents have shown benefits and efficacy from anecdotal or previous experience. Once more data or information about a particular patient's disease process manifests, the empiric regimen is often tailored and titrated to meet the specific needs of that patient according to sensitivity/susceptibility data. Examples of this treatment is the use of a standard dose of antibiotics for pneumonia at its onset, often in emergency room settings. Blood and sputum cultures are drawn only when cultures and sensitivities are available. Only then are antibiotics altered based on culture and sensitivity results.

Prophylaxis Treatment

This methodology is often applied pre-emptively when there is a suspected outbreak or infection. This methodology is designed and used to prevent the disease from occurring.

Pre-Exposure

The dispensing of medication, antibiotics or vaccines prior to occurrence of the disease in anticipation to prevent or mitigate impact. Examples are malaria prophylaxis.

Post-Exposure

Same principles but implemented after the PUI or population has been exposed to an epidemic or a disease. Examples would be taking cipro after there has been anthrax exposure. The line between prophylaxis and post-exposure can often be a thin one, dependent on the suspected level of exposure.

Definitive Treatment

This is your bread-and-butter treatment option, when a clear-cut diagnosis is established by your physician or medical professional. It could be the same regimen or medication which is used for prophylaxis such as cipro for anthrax. Once the disease is confirmed by any diagnostic modality, lab analysis, blood serum, cytology, pathology or radiology, the treatment that ensues as a result is considered definitive treatment.

Concordant Treatment

Empiric therapy is initiated as soon as the samples or cultures are obtained before the treatment is initiated. Once the results of those cultures come back and show that the initial treatment (empiric therapy) regimen initiated is sensitive enough to be effective against the pathogen, empiric therapy starts. These outcome measures reflect better patient prognosis.

Discordant Treatment

The empiric regimen, which was initiated at the outset as the best guess, shows that the regimen was not effective against the organism based on the results of culture and sensitivity. In other words, there was a lack of better kill, portending a trend leaning towards the worst patient outcome. An example is poor survival of community acquired pneumonia if the initial antibiotic regimen is not selected carefully, i.e., based on the antibiogram of that institution or a particular community.

Epidemiology & Statistics

THE BRANCH OR study of medicine dealing with incidence, prevalence, and distribution of disease. Much more involved than merely the study of a single disease, epidemiology looks at various aspects of disease patterns and provides insight into endemics, epidemics and pandemics. Think of it as a high-level macro study to a degree, examining local and global impact of the desired illness. Epidemiology is central in mitigation strategies as well as the classification of the design and control of the disease. Epidemiologists are to thank for large-scale studies of how diseases affect the general public.

Clinical Studies

There are a few central tenants in clinical studies, or research instances that follow the eat-your-vegetables scientific method. There is a hypothesis, evidence, and conclusion, along with refinement and factors that could make the evidence a false positive. Different kinds of clinical studies have varying degrees of impact based on the level of evidence provided by the study methodology. To visualize the hierarchy of the level of evidence provided by these studies, an evidence pyramid is used (See figure below). Studies on the top of the pyramid represent strongest evidence where those at the bottom represent the weakest evidence.

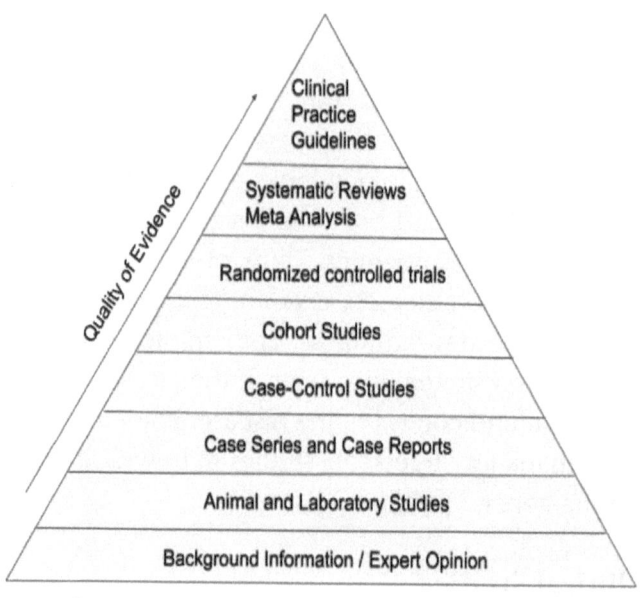

Types of Studies

Generally, the higher up you are on the pyramid, the better your quality of evidence will be.

Anecdotes, Editorials, Ideas, Opinions (AEIO)

Although AEIO lie at the bottom of our evidence pyramid, ideas, opinions, and anecdotes can serve a valuable purpose. Although our friends may be little more than an untested "Wabi-Sabi" set of ideas seemingly without study designs or tangibility to real world events, AEIO can be the bedrock of a surprise medical breakthrough. Our friends can be considered like a nursery of stars before the formation of the sun if you will, amorphous and imperfect but surprisingly vital.

Case Reports and Case Series

A case report is an observational study that describes findings from a single patient with a disease or condition. There is no comparison group. Case reports often describe a rare condition or rare intervention with optimistic results. They may offer important clinical insights or clues at the risk of being misleading. Case *series* offer a slightly higher level of evidence compared to case *reports*. Case *reports* describe an event where patients all receive the same intervention. As with a case report, there is no control group. The study population is often ill-defined. Most case *series* are not consecutive (inviting strong selection bias) or population-based (impeding generalizability).

Cross-Sectional Studies

A cross-sectional study involves looking at data from a population at one specific point in time. The participants in this type of study are selected based on particular variables of interest. They are observational studies and cannot be used to determine the cause of a disease. This type of research can be used to describe characteristics that exist in a community, but not to determine cause-and-effect relationships between the variables.

Case-Control Studies

This is a statistical study that compares 2 groups of individuals, one *with* the disease (cases) with the one *without* the disease (control). This type of study is usually done to study the outcome of a rare disease.

Cohort Studies

This is a statistical term describing groups of people or study groups. In the research literature, it implies the study of a disease to establishing a link between the cause of the disease and the outcomes.

PROSPECTIVE

A longitudinal study that moves "forward in time" to look at a disease or intervention. For example, data pertaining to morbidity and mortality related to patients with treated versus untreated sleep apnea. The patients with OSA are observed over time, moving forward or prospectively, to determine and observe these outcomes. The Framingham Heart Health Study is also such an example of a prospective longitudinal study.

RETROSPECTIVE
This is observational research looking "back in time" to see archival data. It examines the data to assess what factors were responsible for a certain outcome, between various groups with and without intervention. This could be a case control, case series or cohort study. Even though the level of evidence in a retrospective study is weaker than that of *prospective* study, "retro" studies serve a very important purpose in identifying risk factors like diseases and medications, in treated and untreated groups.

Confounding Variable
A single or a group of factors, which may imply an association, but is not a true determinant of cause and effect. For example, moderate alcohol consumption was once labelled as a cause of lung cancer. However, once a detailed statistical analysis was conducted, the report revealed that the true association was cigarette smoking, which was often accompanied with alcohol consumption. The study revealed that people who smoked also drank alcohol and had a higher incidence of lung cancer. Thus, drinking was the confounding variable.

Blinding in clinical research studies
A statistical term used in the conduct of research studies, where various aspects of the study and execution of research techniques are not revealed to the investigators. In other words, concealment of a group allocation from one or more individuals. Blinding typically helps reduce various types of biases that may emerge in the study.

SINGLE BLINDED
One member of the team is blinded. This could be the principal investigator, study site, or statistician.

DOUBLE BLINDED
Pick any two of the above and conceal the study details or any aspect of the data.

Allocation Concealment
This is a statistical term applied as to how the experimental drug or intervention is handled. Usually, it is hidden from either the principal investigator, site coordinators and or patients. This strategy reduces the level of bias, which may have detrimental effects if details or specifics of the drug or intervention are known.

Randomized Control Trials
A statistical term applied to a clinical trial, where true representatives of the population are included

for studies. There are various methods involved in the randomization process which gives an optimal opportunity to the *people living in the community* to be part of the intervention or study. Often this is used generically, at other times it is specified or further delineated, for example: females in certain age groups. Many randomized control trials were performed in the research and development process of COVID-19 vaccine launch.

Meta-Analysis-Review Studies

This is one of the strongest research tools available as it is a combination of various studies, randomized controlled studies, and review articles.

Retrospective Studies

A statistical term applied to studies conducted with information already available. Think of Marty McFly formulating a conclusion with his extensive knowledge of the past. This kind of study is inherently weaker because researchers do not have much control of the variables. No intervention can be applied, as the events have already occurred.

Prospective Studies

A study design where a drug or intervention is studied for the future. In stark opposition to the retrospective studies, this study design is much more powerful, albeit expensive, as data points and subjects are continuously analyzed. Researchers have a lot of control here, where outcomes can be closely controlled, and intervention of study can be halted for both early positive or negative outcomes.

Null Hypothesis
Used in study or hypothesis generation. The concept states to essentially "prove yourself wrong." For example, if the theory is that drug X influences a particular disease hypothesis, then the null hypothesis would be that drug X doesn't have the proposed effect on *that* disease, which is being studied or investigated.

Correlation Study
A type of study examining the correlation or coincidence of another factor in disease occurrence. For example, the incidence of lung cancer in the United States correlated over a certain period of time to cheese production. Even though these two data points line up quite linearly to each other, studies don't reveal a causation between the two sets.

Type I Error
Basically a sort of false positive. Let's say you have a null hypothesis that seemingly disproves your study. However, a type I error is like a red herring in a detective show, throwing your guess at the killer's identity into frustrating disarray. In other words, this error introduces a serious flaw in the study. Therefore, if a

type I error exists, the results can obviously become scrambled, as can your outcomes. Data extrapolation becomes fuzzy. Just remember: your study + wrong null hypothesis = a type I error.

Type II Error
A statistical term referred to as the "False Negative." This is quite the opposite of type-I error, when the null hypothesis is not rejected aka "error of omission."

Types of Biases in the research studies and analytics

Selection Bias:
The most common flavor of bias, mostly encountered during surveys or polls. Let's say your survey has an inappropriate or wrong sample. You are not going to get accurate and causational results. Election polls love treating the opinions of a narrow set of people as the general sentiment of the entire United States population. This can be done intentionally or unintentionally.

Confirmation Bias:
An inherent bias, when evaluators or analysts know about an outcome and knowingly or unknowingly extract the data to prove that preconceived notion. For example, thinking that all left-handed people are geniuses, but only pulling a sample from Harvard for the study.

Outliers:
A kind of bias which skews data because of extreme values. For example, patients who are 110 years old or have one million dollars in their savings account. These data points are far from the average value in the whole.

Overfitting and Underfitting Bias:
This bias creeps in when data is unvalidated. This can either result in oversimplification or overcomplexity in your data set. Hence, your outcome analysis or the data itself becomes invalid. Over assumption is treated as the true outcome when it is not.

Confounding Bias:
A "third party" factor which may co-exist but does not cause a desired effect. For example, smoking is correlated with lung cancer, true cause and effect. However, excessive cheese consumption is just a confounding variable in the study of lung cancer and not a true cause.

Statistical Terminology

p-Value
The alpha level set to determine statistical differences in the results achieved in the study. Usually set at <0.05.

Incidence
A statistical term which indicates the new onset of disease. For example, the incidence of COVID-19 virus in the USA.

Prevalence
The presence of a particular disease in a region or country. For example, prevalence of TB in the Sub-Saharan region.

Sensitivity aka PID (Positive in Disease)
A statistical term which signifies a positive test in a diseased person. An example of a sensitive test is the

PPD or TB test, which is conducted to screen masses in high-risk populations, or an annual PPD test in healthcare workers. This test is done with an intent to treat. If the person tests positive and doesn't have the disease, it's called a "False Positive."

Specificity aka NIH (Negative In Health)
A "false negative." The test reads negative, but the person in actuality has the disease. This is a statistical binary term.

Positive Predictive Value - PPV
A statistical term implying that a person who tested positive truly has the disease being investigated. Hence it reduces false positive tests.

Negative Predictive Value - NPV
A statistical term implying that a person who tested negative in fact doesn't have the disease. Hence it reduces the false negative test.

Relative Risk Reduction - RRR
A term referring to how much reduction in the illness occurred in the treatment group as compared with the cohort or placebo. RRR is a study in the efficacy of a specific treatment. Relative Risk Reduction of 0.8 means 20% risk reduction in the treatment group. If there is no change in the outcome, RRR will be 0.0 or 0%.
RRR 100% × (1 − RR).

Absolute Risk Reduction - ARR
A statistical term referring to the risk of developing a disease or specific side effect over a period of time or as a result of medication or intervention. For example, the risk of developing heart disease over the lifespan of a certain individual could be 10% or 0.1%.

Numbers to Needed to Treat - NTT
A statistical term which helps determine the power of the study. In other words, this is done to assess how many subjects will be needed to find statistical significance. Absolute risk reduction is calculated to see how many patients need to be treated to have a certain risk of adverse event or complication. For example, how many patients need to be treated to see potential benefits vs. the risk of bleeding in patients receiving *tPA*. This is calculated before any study or intervention is done for research purposes.

Numbers to Harm - NNH
This is opposite to numbers to treat. This implies how many patients will be harmed for a patient to benefit from the intervention.

Confidence Interval - CI
A statistical term depicting the range of values within 95% certainty where the true value of the entire population lies. Since it is impossible to study the entire population, a small but representative sample of the

population is studied. The results inferred from that small group are accurately reflective of the entire population.

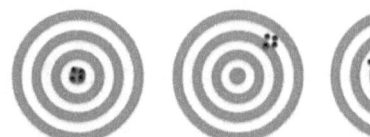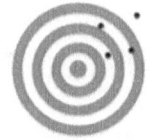

(anonymous-n.d)

A-Accurate *aka Precise aka Bullseye*
A statistical term describing a test or treatment which is accurate (valid) and precise (reliable). This should score a perfect Bullseye on the plot.

B-Precision *aka Reliability*
A statistical term describing a test or treatment which is reliable but may not be accurate. This will correspond to a hole close to each other, but away from the bullseye.

C-Accuracy *aka Validity*
A statistical term which describes the accuracy of a test or treatment. And accurate test or treatment will be considered a valid one. This is like getting your darts within one or two circles of the bull's eye. Less than perfect, but still ideal.

D-Neither Accurate nor Precise *aka Not Valid-Not Reliable*
A statistical description of data or an outcome measure, about as accurate as scattered buckshot littering your dartboard. This outcome cannot be relied upon.

Statistical Tests - commonly and frequently used

CHI SQUARE - $x2$
This statistical term tests the relationship between categorical variables, assessing whether the variables are related or independent. It also helps determine if the difference between observed expected data is due to chance, or due to a correlational or causational relationship between the variables under study.

STUDENT T-TEST
This test calculates the difference between the two means. The greater the vastness of the t-test, the greater the evidence *against* the null hypothesis.

MANN-WHITNEY U TEST AKA MANN WHITNEY WILCOXON TEST
This test compares the difference in the *means* of two tests, when the dependent variables are either nominal or continuous. It tests whether two samples come from the same population. It compares two groups of population, treatments, or conditions.

Statistical Presentation of data

KAPLAN MEIER CURVE

A graphical representation of survival extracted from lifetime data. It shows the survivability of a group of people over time after an intervention and is typically compared with the cohort of the untreated group. Simply calculated by dividing the number of patients that survived as compared with the patients at risk or untreated.

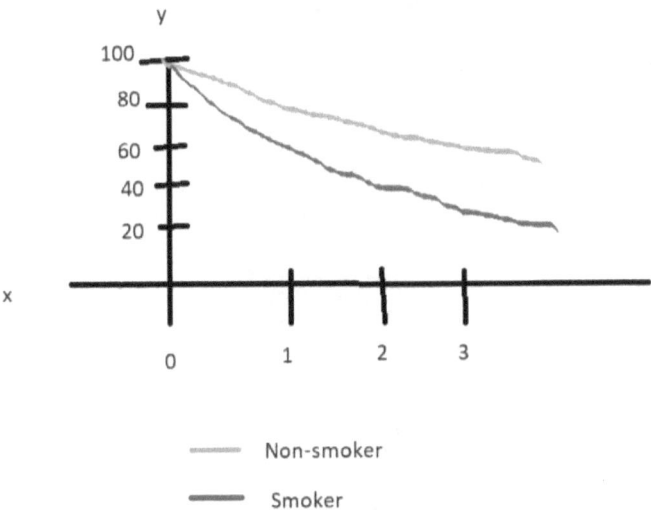

(Shahwar Abbasi)

Pie Graph or Pie Chart

A type of graph that shows data in a circular fashion. Each variable is represented as a pie slice or a wedge. This usually represents categorical variables. It shows the relative contribution (slice or a pie) in a total which is the entire circle. It illustrates numerical proportions.

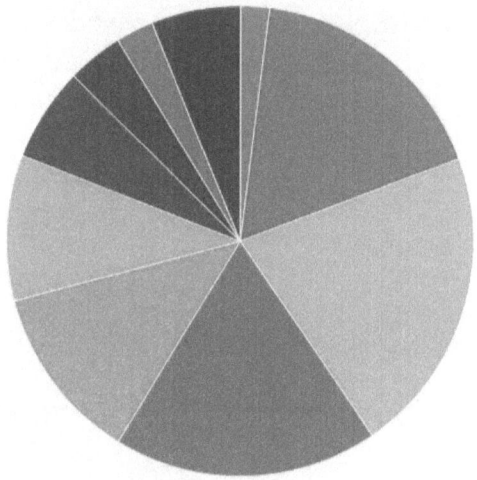

(anonymous-n.d)

Bar-Graph aka Bar Chart

A data representation in the form of vertical bars. Usually, the height and color represent the data points, which can be compared visually. It is a great tool for graphical representation of financial data. It can present data, quantities, and numbers.

STATISTICAL TERMINOLOGY

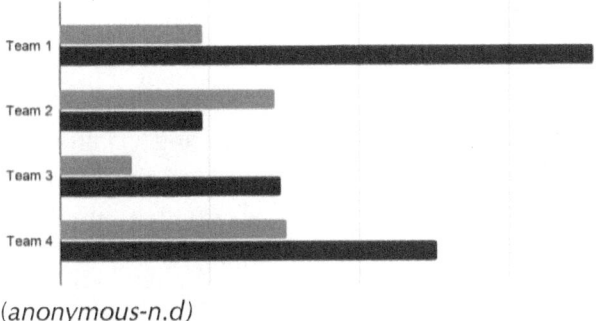

(anonymous-n.d)

SCATTER PLOT OR SCATTER GRAPH

A graphical representation of the mathematical data of variables represented as dots. Each data point and its position present a value on the x or y axis. One can observe relationships between various variables. The scatter plot is inferred as positive, negative or none as there is no correlation.

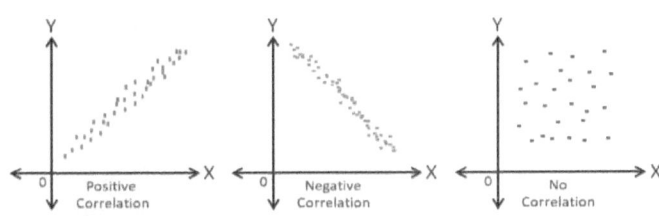

(anonymous-n.d)

Types of Statistical Data

Linear
Usually presented as a graph depicting continuous variables over time. The data points are arranged sequentially, connecting current data points to the later ones in a linear or sequential manner.

Non-Linear Data
A graph depicting continuous variables over time. The data points are arranged sequentially, connecting a current data point to the next one in a linear or sequential manner.

Index Case
Often referred to as "patient zero," an index case is a statistical and epidemiologic term that defines the first case associated with an endemic epidemic. This is often attributed to infected cases of communicable disease.

Mortality Rate
A term describing the number of deaths during a specified period in a particular population, due to a specific cause or disease. It is described either as a percentage or in 100,000, or occasionally in millions when the mortality rate is relatively low.

Case Fatality Ratio
The mortality associated with the disease. For example, the CFR due to Lassa fever is 23%, which is a lot higher as compared with that of COVID-19, which is about 2%.

Incidence
Occurrence of a new disease in a specific area. This is an emergence or outbreak of an infection or a disease.

Prevalence
Presence of a particular disease in a specific region, i.e., Ebola in West Africa (Guinea, Liberia, Sierra Leone).

Apex
This represents the highest number of cases or the climax of the disease. In other words, the apex is when the disease is at its peak. This represents a specific time frame, for example, the infectivity rate of the Flu virus during winter months.

Asymptomatic Carrier State
Connotes a person who is infected but doesn't exhibit symptoms of the disease. However, that person can be contagious and can potentially spread the disease to other people or animals. When tested, these individuals test positive for the disease but don't exhibit any signs or symptoms of the disease. These asymptomatic

carriers play a major role in the spread of disease during epidemics and pandemics. Since they often go unrecognized as they are not diagnosed with the disease, they do not use appropriate preventive quarantine measures during acute points of the disease.

Community Spread
The existence and spread of disease in a particular community, city, county, or state. This analysis is critical in the identification of the geographic location or group of people affected by a given disease, so preventive and mitigation strategies can be implemented.

Epidemic aka "Outbreak"
Per the CDC, the occurrence of more cases of disease than expected in a given area or specific group of people over a particular period of time. Simply put, it's a rapid progression of a communicable disease that occurs in a short span of time. It is usually exceeding expectations or calculations of the disease projection.

Epidemic Patterns

POINT SOURCE EPIDEMIC
Epidemics that emanate from a single source. They tend to spike during a short period followed by a slow decline. A perfect example is an outbreak of cholera or hepatitis A. Transmission is often person to person.

Common Source Epidemics
A pattern of epidemic when multiple people or a group of people get infected from the same source.

Progressive or Propagated Epidemics
Person to person spread of infection.

Mixed Epidemics
A pattern showing a combination of both point or common outbreaks with propagation. For example, typhoid fever.

Source-Contact Tracing
A technique to trace the source responsible for the spread of a given disease. Researchers usually start with the known first or index case, and they continue to follow the progression from person to person spread. Researchers look for patterns of spread of the virus or bacteria in an infected person or animal.

Antigenic Variation
Referring to how a single virus can exhibit variable cross reactivity, when tested with a standard laboratory serum *in-vitro* (testing in the lab environment or outside the body of a living being, animal or human).

Antigenic Drift
Subtle changes or mutations in the antigenic properties of a given virus. This results in the changes

in the numbers associated with "H" and "N." It is a slow change and therefore can maintain its antigenic property while still being capable of mounting an immune-mediated antibody response. These changes are a common occurrence, which continue to occur throughout the replication process of the virus's life cycle. The "progeny" of the virus still closely resemble the genetic code of its "ancestor." This change results in host antibodies capable of recognizing the antigenic glycogens and mounting an immune response, a phenomenon called "cross protection."

Sometimes *drift* can be so profound that many times a given virus mutates to the point that it drives an old vaccine obsolete. Another example is multiple episodes of flu infection in the same season. Coronavirus doesn't have the predilection for either antigenic shift or drift as compared with the flu virus.

Antigenic Shift

Shift, on the other hand, implies a rather abrupt change in antigenic properties. Only certain species of virus can shift with more than one genetic 'cassette.' Influenza, for example, has eight genes. If different flu strains mix or match, an entire gene can be replaced, causing a new subtype radically different from its predecessors. This process occurs frequently with zoonotic infection, where a shift may be needed to jump to another species. Antigenic shifts are more closely related to epidemics and pandemics because immunity to prior strains often is unaffected against shifts.

Pandemic Shifts

You won't find this term in an official capacity, but there is still some validity in its occurrence. This theory is sort of like the oft-heard preservation of matter theory. It basically says that endemic or pandemic diseases didn't simply disappear, but shift to a different region, hop a geographical boundary if you will, and head to a new populace.

One example is TB, which was once prevalent in the Western hemisphere, but has found a new home in developing countries. It was a change in patient's nutrition, and an overall shift towards a public health scheme focusing on sanitation that largely kicked the disease out of America, even though there was a slight uptick in the incidence of TB in the West after HIV/AIDS became a novel disease.

Today, the concept of pandemic shift presents a near daily change of nomenclature. TB can be someone's novel coronavirus, while for the west, it almost becomes a romanticized memory.

Pandemic Resurgence-Recurrence

When thinking about a pandemic resurgence, think of the black death. Each time the black death visited humanity as a large-scale event, it returned with seemingly greater ferocity, or *vengeance* if you are a fan of anthropomorphizing. Around 50-60% of Europe's population was annihilated due to the black death, but even after taking half, it came back, wiping a city here, a port there. This resurgence theory sits pretty with the concept that pandemics turn to endemic diseases when controlled. However, the threat of mutation may always be present.

Antigenic Divergence

Also referred to as antigenic variation or antigenic alteration, this avoidance and protective mechanism of a virus or bacterium which causes alteration in its protein or carbohydrate moiety. This structural makeup is used to protect the organism to mount the appropriate immunologic response. By gaining the opportunity to alter or vary its structural component by substitution of the structural component, these organisms remain elusive and hence avoid damaging effects of the host immune-mediated killing. Thus, antigenic heterogeneity renders the microbes more pathogenic and deadly.

Antigenic Stasis

A genetically quiescent period, when the structural integrity and phenotypical characteristics of a virus remain fairly stable over the course of its evolution. The genetic sequence of a virus remains neutral. This could be a period of its reparative process, or before or after any amino acid sequence changes or alterations.

Antigenic Evolution

A phenomenon where viruses can evolve into new strains. As a result of this evolution, each subsequent mutated strain or progeny varies its phenotypical behavior, rendering it protected from antimicrobial agents.

Genetic Viral Diversity

When various viruses of distant features have been prevalent in specific areas, there could be low genetic diversity, which implies infection by a single event or multiple events of viruses, which share similar characteristics. Examples are H1N1 viruses.

Genetic and Racial Diversity

Contrasting genetic viral diversity, this term refers to the diverse racial and genetic makeup of humans either offering a perfect breeding ground for virus proliferation or a stark resistance. Examples are smallpox, a common childhood ailment amongst Europeans, which decimated nearly 90% of the Aztec population. Another example is how the Sickle Cell trait offered protection to the African population against malaria, while causing a significant shift in morbidity and mortality in African descendants living in the Americas and Europe. COVID-19 also showed a predilection for Mediterranean genes and other biological attributes, while having a more limited toll in in other populations. These factors are still under immense discussion and research.

Gain of Function

In biological science, where a virus or a virulent pathogen is allowed to replicate in various animal species and is tailored by scientists to induce change its genetic moiety to capture its full virulent potential. While this is a tool to study pathogens in a controlled setting, the worst-case scenario (hypothesized by some as the source of COVID-19 setting) is that gain of function is used to bring out the deadliest mutations of a virus for purposes of total war. As many movies have hypothesized, gain of function can also be used to wipe out certain entire races of people when a virus is tailored for a certain genetic code. Perverse thinking indeed.

Endemic illness

A disease indigenous to a particular geographical area. For example, malaria is endemic to Africa and Asia. Some diseases start spreading under the guise of endemic but become pandemics in the long run. Some diseases do the opposite, starting as a pandemic, but becoming limited to one geographical area or people when the dust settles.

Pandemic disease

When an epidemic spreads beyond its original confines and spreads rapidly across multiple geographical areas, it is called a pandemic.

Epicenter
This term is borrowed from a geological term, which relates to a point on earth's surface which is located vertically above the area of seismic activity. Similarly, in epidemiology this term implies the "hot zone" or "ground zero," of an epidemic or pandemic.

Person Under Investigation - PUI
A unique epidemiological term referring to any person who is suspected to have contracted the disease, either by exposure or contact. This person remains under investigation, surveillance or under quarantine until more information is known. The duration of such isolation depends on the incubation period of the disease or epidemic under investigation.

Confirmed Case
Once the person who was the *Person Under Investigation* (PUI), is confirmed positive for that particular disease or infection, they are referred to as a confirmed case.

Harm Reduction
A group of strategies which reduce or mitigate the deleterious effects of a disease or behavior. The principle is that a behavior or disorder is hard to eliminate. For example, intravenous drug abuse is common and in certain areas is inevitable, therefore clean needles are disposable.

Vectors
A Vector is typically a biting insect or tick that has the capability of transmitting diseases across various species. Bats acting as a vector transmitting COVID-19 infection is a classic example of a vector-borne illness. The mosquito is another common vector for malaria and Zika virus, while white tail deer tick are vectors for Lyme disease. Rodents and bats are usually the reservoirs of many diseases and are considered some of the most senior vectors. Vectors usually carry diseases without displaying symptoms themselves, a bad deal for everyone else.

Biological Host
An animal or plant as a dwelling place for a virus. The perfect host allows for peak nutrition and nourishment for the virus's growth and replication.

Host Classification:
Accidental Host: an unconventional host that the parasite does not use.
Incidental Host: hosts the parasite as the final site and doesn't transmit it further.
Reservoir Host: helps sustain the parasite in its quiescent or non-infective stage.
Primary Host: the final or definitive host.

Host Factors:
Certain traits in the host species that make it more susceptible i.e., genetic factors or disease, etc.
Intermediate Host:
This host helps in the asexual maturation of the host.
Definitive Host (Final Host):
This host helps complete the sexual stage of the infective organism or the parasite.

Zoonotic Spillover and Transmissibility aka *Host Jumping*
Transmission of a disease from animals to humans. This transmissibility can occur via direct contact such as contact with infected secretion or tissues i.e., rabies

from a rabid dog bite, or indirectly such as air-borne illnesses like the flu. Sometimes, vectors like mosquitoes or ticks play a role in the transmission of the disease.

Biological Warfare-Bioterrorism
The use of biological agents to advance political or military objectives. Historical examples have been reported to include intentional efforts to spread the bubonic plague into Europe during the Middle Ages by Mongolians, catapulting plague victim bodies over the walls of Caffa in 1347. Whether these efforts bore fruit or were counterproductive are best left to a history book. Extensive research and development into bioterrorism and biological warfare occurred throughout the early part of the cold war and is now banned by international treaties. However, there exists a persistent concern that non-state actors will use these agents to great avail, like Bruce Edwards Ivins killing 17 people with mail-in Anthrax in 2001.

Prevention
The most important aspect of curtailing the spread of disease before its occurrence. Preventive measures should be universal in scale to be the most effective. This concept is not unique to new styles of healthcare. Blood or any kind of bodily secretions can be considered infectious, and therefore a commonsense approach to prevention is always necessary. There are various means to achieve these goals, by wearing

disposable gloves or garments to use more sophisticated apparel i.e., hazmat suits and respirators. This is where researchers should brainstorm ways of stopping the disease before it spreads.

Diagnosing an Epidemic

TESTING

BASIC METABOLIC PANEL
Various methods of testing can be applied to the diagnosis and tracing of an epidemic. These tests should ideally be cheap, easily performable and sensitive. Examples are testing air samples for blood, fluids and tissues testing by Enzymatic Linked Immunoassay (ELISA), Polymerase Chain Reaction (PCR). Biopsy and tissue analysis can be applied based on virology or microbiology principles.

ANTIGEN TEST
This test determines the presence of viral antigen or components. It has a rather quick turnaround time and tends to have high sensitivity but lower specificity. Therefore, it is often used as a screening tool.

ANTIBODY TEST
Performed by detecting the chemical reaction of the test subject, compared to that of a positive

control. The test may reveal antibodies i.e., IgM (evidence of recent infection or immunity induced by a vaccine) or IgG (evidence of remote or past infection).

Contact Tracing
The study of contacts who may be related to the spread of infection or disease. This helps in determination of the cause, pattern of disease, spread and treatment modalities. This exhaustive work is achieved by:

>Contact identification
>Contact listing
>Contact follow up

Multiple tools like cell-mobile phone applications have exploded and are being utilized across the world to trace the activities of travelers, including tracing disease back to specific locations, as well as to monitor people under quarantine.

Cluster of Disease
The incidence of an unusually high conglomeration of a particular disease, within a short span of time in a specific geographical location.

Critical Supplies
With every new epidemic and pandemic comes new challenges. Researchers have the tremendous job of

anticipating preventive measures and being prepared for what's to come. A severe stalemate as of the writing of this book, clear and available supply chains should be a part of any emergency preparedness of any country, state or city. Once the outbreak is underway, as we are seeing, there is not nearly enough time, or enough resources to declutter a bottle-necked supply chain. Dwindling supplies can put a burden on the healthcare system, small and large communities, as well as entire countries to boot. The best solution to this problem is the dreaded mantra from *Cobra Kai*. Strike first. "Peacetime" is the ideal time to prepare, anticipate and formulate a mitigation plan before catastrophe hits.

Personal Protective Equipment (PPE)
Gloves
Masks
Respirators
PAPR (Powered Air Pressure Respirator)
Haz-mat suits
Boots
Protective eye equipment and glasses
Donning and doffing practices and guidelines
Decontamination (decon) techniques, zones and protocols

Masks
An umbrella term that represents a face covering, or a fastening which covers the face and mouth. It ranges

from hand-made cloth masks to surgical and N-95 masks. Masks differ in the protection they offer. For example, surgical and cloth masks prevent the spread of the common cold to other vital airborne pathogens in an otherwise healthy person. However, to achieve a specific degree of protection, i.e., health care workers who are directly exposed to TB, or deadly viral pathogens COVID-19, N-95 or higher level masks are recommended. The "95" in N-95 purports 95% protection against particulates, which are 3 micros or higher. The "N" connotes NIOSH (National Institute of Occupational Safety and Health.

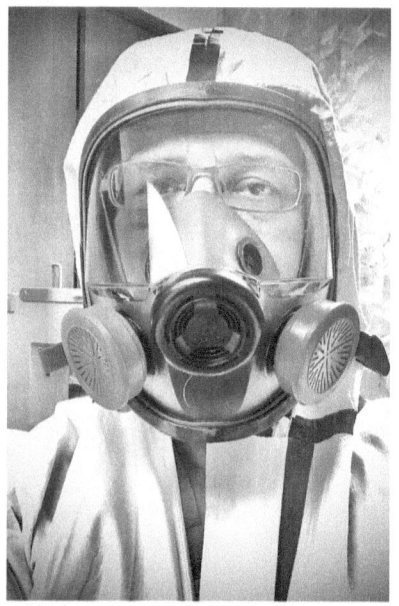

Dr. Anwar treating patients at the height of the pandemic.

Respirators
An enhanced protective device, which offers near 100% protection against any droplet or airborne pathogen and particulate matter. These can be analogue or motor devices, such as PAPR (Powered Air Pressure Respirator) popularized in movies depicting epidemics i.e., *Contagion*.

Ventilators
Equipment meant to provide lifesaving ventilatory and oxygen support to patients with respiratory failure. Ventilators can be invasive, i.e., those introduced into the throat into the trachea "windpipe" and are commonly used in an ICU setting, and non-invasive which can be used both in the hospital and home, i.e., CPAP, AVAPS or BiPAP devices. Non-invasive ventilators often have a mask interface. The majority of these devices are reserved for providing either ventilatory, oxygen or both.

Universal Precautions
Treating blood, secretions and biological content to be infectious and hazardous.

Vigorous hand washing and decontamination techniques should be exercised when there is an exposure to blood, secretions, and biological content.

Triage Decisions

The triage system was first introduced during the French Revolution, which entailed a system of patient care and source allocation according to the best utilization of available resources. This tool of decision making is not based on the severity of illness, rather it encompasses equitable distribution of resources when the balance of distribution is weighed against it. Basically, it's an exercise protocol to see how best to distribute limited resources and (wo)manpower. Examples of this concept have often been applied in "military triage" where a unique terminology lies in place. Remember that iconic D-Day scene from *Saving Private Ryan*, where the senior medic was walking down the row of injured soldiers to inspect them? One of the words he used was "expectant," or not salvageable, while examining a particularly injured patient. Expectant status is reserved for a gratuitous injury; a bleed or injury that is expected to kill the patient. In this common battlefield situation, especially in World War II, medics would have chosen to not use their valuable resources to save that quickly expiring patient. More salvageable cases, however are referred to as "immediate," while milder cases, or cases of psychological trauma (not to downplay psychology) are termed "delayed."

Similar nomenclature is needed in the environment in which this book is being written. Resources are scarce, and healthcare environments are dynamic to a fault. The basic framework needed to achieve preparedness is to have surge planning and comprehensive inventory of the vital equipment, i.e., ventilators, ICU beds, supplies and staffing. Establishment of command & control and some sort of organizational chart are necessary to cement a very clear line of communication and chain of command.

Collaboration is essential between administration and clinical staff, with a spill-over assistance system in place with the help of a local command and control police: the fire department, city, state and federal governments.

More than just a plan of action for a grave scenario, triage has great power to spawn policies and procedures regarding rotating call schedules and install appropriate allocation of available resources to front line workers, including PPE. More high level and long-term policy changes of triage can also be designing or revising patient care according to the standard of care, the patient's family engagement, healthcare worker support with logistics and end of life policies.

Probably the most challenging triage examples are the high requirement of ventilators and ECMO (Extracorporeal Membrane Oxygenation) during the outbreaks of H1N1 and COVID-19.

There may be some instinctual barriers to allocating more resources to those patients who are in better shape than someone in dire need of treatment. The sickest of the patients often require most attention and source utilization, many times when there are not enough resources to go around. This tough scenario warrants appropriate bedside decision, where efforts should be focused on the salvageable cases to minimize inefficient use of limited resources. Ideally, one would apply the lean six sigma principles. Other triage challenges include ethics, emotions of the healthcare provider, preconceived notions about the disease and even medicolegal issues. Here's to you, pesky lawyers!

Herd Immunity *aka*
"Herd Effect"
"Community Immunity"
"Population Immunity"
"Social Immunity"

It is difficult for a disease to spread, no matter how contagious, within an immune population. This kind of immunity can also render an indirect form of protection to non-immune populations, when a large group of the immune population is either vaccinated or is infected prior. Developing and dispensing a safe and effective vaccine is the preferred way to get herd immunity by a mile as opposed to attempting what an alarming chunk of the population refers to as natural immunity through infection. Attempting natural immunity through infection and developing antibodies as sequela is a nasty and random process. Untreated diseases do what they do best, causing significant morbidity and mortality in patients with any underlying chronic disease, cancer or immunocompromised status.

The transmissibility of any given disease affects the ability of a population to incur immune status. Transmissibility is usually measured as R0 (pronounced R naught), the number of persons an infected person is likely to pass disease to. Herd immunity is typically associated with effective immunity in a proportion of the population equal to $1-1/R0$, meaning that a highly transmissible virus like measles, with an R0 of 12, requires near universal vaccination, while a more typical virus, like SARS-CoV-2, may require 70% of people to have effective immunity. With a vaccine that is 70% effective, that would require 100% of people to be immunized; a 95% effective vaccine would require closer to 75%.

Immune-compromised Host (ICH)

This represents the population of patients with reduced, altered, or impaired immune systems. This group consists of patients who have cancer, are being treated with immune modulating drugs for chemotherapy, or connective tissue disease. Patients who are taking high dose steroids >20 mg of prednisone for prolonged periods of time i.e., months to years, are also included in this category. This section also includes another subgroup of individuals who have diabetes, heart diseases and chronic pro-inflammatory conditions, where immunity is not as robust with as their healthy counterparts. This subgroup is more susceptible to certain diseases including bacterial, viral and fungal infections.

Hygiene Hypothesis

A controversial hypothesis based on the claim that if someone is born in a small and affluent household condition, and birth order, that they have less susceptibility to get infections or allergies. Exposure to certain infections and allergic mediators renders the host protection to the deleterious effects later in life and hence establishes immune tolerance to that particular disease or allergic manifestation. It's more applicable in more temperate climatic diseases such as *Helicobacter Pylori* or Hepatitis A. Atopic allergies, asthma and cytokine mediated processes are also implicated in this hypothesis.

Germ Theory of Disease

The basis of this theory is that various microorganisms, viruses, bacteria and fungi cause certain diseases. During the turn of the century, the germ theory was solidified, with findings that stated germs were the root cause of infectious disease. Dr. Josephine Baker championed that concept early on and implemented various efforts in the early 1900's to mitigate the spread of disease and establish preventative measures. With the critical invention of penicillin, many treatment modalities also came to light.

Epidemics and Societal Impact

Strong inferences are taken from *Epidemics and Society* by Professor Snowden. He describes various epidemics and the impact on societies of that particular era in history. One of the main chapters discusses "The Sanitary Movement," and how it revolutionized patient care in France and England.

Population and Disease

This branch of health science deals with the impact of disease on the population and vice versa i.e., the effects of population on various diseases. Diabetes for example is a disease with specific implications on some parts of a general population. However, examining specific disease effects on certain populations becomes tricky and fast changing during an event like COVID-19. The history of endemics and pandemics usually always occur in a close-knit people-livestock setting. Such outbreaks rarely occur in isolated and sparsely populated areas, like the Amazon jungle. It is a concentrated population that engages in trade and travel that leads to the spread of disease.

Fear Factor - Fear of Unknown

The fear of the unknown is a phenomenon plaguing humanity since the days of Cain, Abel and Seth. More than just the handful of short-term symptoms like shortness of breath and quickened heart rate, the fear of the unknown can be described as a persistent and embedded human state of being or ontological state. This fear of the unknown takes many manifestations, especially during such a generational event like COVID-19. People start asking questions like "will this pandemic ever go away?" Many times, the fear of the unknown settles into other parts of human lifestyle, including poorer driving, or lashing out against Asian Americans for Trump's abhorrent "Chinese Virus" moniker for the disease. The fear of the unknown creeps into society and lawmaker's habits at large as well, with back-and-forth mask mandates issued by the CDC, and economic pivoting by small and large businesses. Some days, the masks were off, and other days, the masks were on. This is another battlefield entirely.

The fear of the unknown is a paradox in some sense, as it pertains to the new pandemic. The fear of the unknown is a daily driver for the average human, a constant state of being, if you will. Only when something like a deadly pandemic is thrown into the mix, does the short-term existential worry start pouring out of every orifice like a fire hydrant bursting at the seams.

Nothing screamed this condition more than the toilet paper shortage at the start of the pandemic. The fear of reaching for nothing after deploying a number two seemed to send shockwaves of uncertainty through the general populace, often more so than the worry of masking up.

This fear of the unknown continued to hammer dents into the supply chain, with PPE, medicines and equipment bottlenecked for healthcare workers, let alone the average American. Let's put a label on this, shall we? Although you won't find "The TP Phenomenon" in the Merriam Webster, we think that it serves as a great capstone on this outrageous phenomenon.

Treatment Modalities
Although these epidemics are textbook cataclysm, they offer an ample opportunity for but offer an opportunity for nuances in pharmaceutical R&D and the utilization of experimental medications. One such experimental and developing program is Telehealth, which was in a stage of infancy before the pandemic. When CMS approved an ICD-10 code for such services, telehealth really came onto its own. Facetime and other smartphone features were often the only line of communication between the outside world and the ICU when the threat of extreme spread axed visitation rights by a significant margin. I have experienced too many instances where an iPhone screen was the last place families saw or talked to their departing loved ones.

Vaccines
Vaccines consist of biological moieties that have similar antigenic components as that of the same virus that causes the disease to begin with. These antigens are extracted from the virus and carefully killed and

weakened, so it is no longer antigenic but has the protein component which is perceived by the host as an antigen and an antibody response is mounted. Vaccines have been used as far back as Feb 5, 1777, the date when George Washington himself mandated variolation, the precursor of current day vaccines. The entire American force was protected against smallpox, as disease and attrition are some of the greatest killers on the battlefield. The American military and military schools are not shy from issuing vaccine mandates. However, in the age of Facebook dogma, sentiment is shifting against this age-old technique. Heck. even those in the Ming Dynasty, starting around the 14th century, practiced inoculation as well, the precursor to vaccines, by applying a bit of smallpox sore (yuck) into a breach of the skin. Seems like we have it pretty good these days.

CLASSIFICATION
1- Live Attenuated Vaccines

> Prepared by obtaining and weakening the component of the live virus, which results in an immune-mediated antibody response. Examples include Measles, Mumps, Rubella, Yellow fever, Rota virus, smallpox and chickenpox. Those who shouldn't get these vaccines include patients with compromised immunity, underlying medical conditions, or ones who are taking immune modifying or transplant rejection medication.

2- Inactivated Vaccines

These vaccines contain a killed virus. The immunity rendered by these vaccines is not as robust as that of live attenuated ones, but they provide sufficient dead antigenic components for the host's immune system to generate a defense response. Examples include flu, polio, rabies and hepatitis-A.

3- Recombinant Vaccines

These vaccines are made from a component of the virus, i.e., protein, capsid or sugar. The advantage of the recombinant vaccines is the safety of use regardless of the host's immune system status. Examples include pneumococcal, HiB, Hep B, HPV and shingles.

4- Toxoid Vaccines

These vaccines are made from toxins produced by a given germ. The recipient's immune system produces antibodies against the toxin, rendering it less antigenic. Tetanus and Diphtheria are examples of the toxoid vaccines.

5- RNA Vaccines

This novel method of vaccine biotechnology, developed in the wake of the COVID-19 pandemic. Messenger RNA *(m-rna)* is produced to battle against the antigen contained in the virus. This Messenger RNA produces an antibody response against the virus and hence confers immunity. This unique vaccine is being manufactured by world renowned pharmaceutical company Pfizer and the relatively new kid on the block, MODERNA. Fun fact: the last three letters of the company spell out "RNA".

Although mRNA technology had originated from the prestigious UPenn program, there was little general acceptance from the scientific community. Thankfully however, it found acceptance and widespread use. Although this vaccine variant is challenging to mass produce and store (it must be stored and shelved in a certain temperature for a limited amount of time) this breakthrough biotech has the potential to change medicine as we know it.

5-DNA Vaccines

A novel and powerful method for vaccine research, involving the deliberate introduction into tissues of a DNA plasmid carrying an antigen-coding gene that transfects cells in vivo and results in an immune response. DNA vaccines have several distinct advantages, which include the ease of manipulation, use of a generic technology, simplicity of manufacture, and chemical and biological stability. In addition, DNA vaccines are a great leveler among researchers around the world because they provide unprecedented ease of experimentation.

6-Recombinant Vector Vaccine

Recombinant vector vaccines are live replicating viruses that are engineered to carry extra genes derived from a pathogen. These extra genes produce proteins against the antigens, which generate immunity. These vaccine genomes may evolve to lose extra genes during the manufacturing of the vaccine or replication within an individual. There is also a concern that this evolution might severely limit the vaccine's efficacy.

Antibody Treatment

This treatment modality entails infusion of extracted monoclonal antibodies that can thwart the progression of the disease inside of an infected individual. This antibody response *in-vivo* ensues a cascade of immunomodulating events that protects the cells and organs from the detrimental effects of the virus. The example is *Bamlanivimab* infusion for outpatient treatment of mild to moderate SARS Cov-2 infection.

Convalescent Plasma

A controversial and often ineffective treatment modality. Plasma or serum extracted from patients who previously developed infection and supposedly carry serum rich antibodies to fight off the infection. For example, in the early stages of the COVID-19 pandemic, when no vaccine had been developed, patients who had fully recovered from the infection donated their plasma to be transfused in very sick COVID patients. However, this practice lost favor due to lack of clear benefit, and in some cases, an uptick in potential harm.

Genomic Surveillance

The study and surveillance of various viral strains and genomes, usually employed to study genetic mutations in a particular virus. Usually employed on an ongoing basis to study various strains that emerge yearly such as flu strains, this technique focuses on viruses with rapid transmissibility, i.e., SARS CoV-2 (Covid-19) infection, B.1.1.7 and P.1 strains. This helps retool vaccine manufacturing and modification as needed.

Anti Vaxxers-Vaccine Hesitancy

Oh boy, here we go. It is generally a good thing to not take many things at face value. Like when your uncle Randy who thinks Satan himself is somehow involved in vaccine production. However, we all know that there is a fine line between skepticism and ignorance. The anti vaxxer crusade turns everyone into their own version of Pope Urban II, but even then, perhaps we are overestimating the processing power of these individuals. For those who "want to watch the world burn," a la Nolan, anti vaxxers choose to pay a hefty price, often with the blood of their family and friends.

One of the nastier chapters in the COVID-19 saga, a large segment of the American population is "choosing" not to get vaccinated. Instead, they have been infected with a Stockholm Syndrome, where their captor COVID-19 seems like the better alternative to freedom. Anti vaxxers not only want to become a victim of COVID, but also want to serve as a host body (or viral incubator) for others. Vaccine hesitancy is somewhat acceptable when the risks might be unknown or more common than benefits, however, the worst thing that the COVID-19 vaccine did to me was a dull headache.

Different from COVID anti-vaxxers, general "Anti Vaxxer" may refer to a group of people who are opposed to the administration of vaccines, *period*. Strategies may include a delay in getting a vaccine instead of outright refusal. The most common context of this is when a parent of a school-age child refuses to allow vaccine administration to their child due to social, religious, medical or personal reasons and beliefs. Facebook Dogma is again, our favorite culprit. Reasons for this ontological state include conspiracy theories like vaccines being the epicenter for autism, a "theory" bearing little fruit. COVID anti vaxxers like to point to the reduction of human fertility, which has been linked to teenagers not getting the vaccine, or not getting permission from their parents. You'll be right about something, one of these days, Uncle Randy, but today's probably not the day. We think that Obama is more likely a lizard person from the Alpha Draconis star system.

This general anti vaxxer movement seemingly has no bounds either. Many have started their crusade in south asia, where anti vaxx cells sponsor a burgeoning anti-polio vaccine movement in Pakistan and Afghanistan. This has exacerbated the preexisting polio crisis, hampering WHO and Gates Foundation efforts to eradicate this debilitating childhood illness.

As Mr. Miyagi says, "vax on, vax off..." or something like that. Sorry, I couldn't resist. I am a father, after all.

Public Health Policy vs Public Relations Postures

An organized strategy used by teams consisting of epidemiologists, and state and federal health professionals to find a strategy to mitigate the spread of the disease or epidemic in a specific geographical region. This is an over simplistic definition as there are multiple, regulatory and public health agencies, who partake in this plan, to implement appropriate strategies and make laws.

Psychological Impact

Often the most criminally overlooked yet important aspects of public health and anthropology is the psychological impact of a pandemic. The feeling of helplessness and loss of control plays a major role in the etiology of this cluster. The shelter in place order, and the beehive of conflicting politics and information can spawn truly weird psychological manifestations in the general populace. These effects can be empirically prevented or mitigated by a joint task force, both at healthcare and community level.

Biological Warfare

A nasty occurrence where the attacker uses virulent pathogens, bacteria or other such toxins against an opposing military force, or against the general populace in a terror-style attack. A primary lesson in the study of warfare is familiarizing oneself with the basics of the Chemical, Biological, Radiological and Nuclear (CBRN) impact, both militarily, strategically and psychologically. True terror is felt when on there is a bio-terror attack on civilians, like dirty bombs or the sarin gas attack in the Tokyo railway system. Physical damage is one thing, but there is also the desired psychological breakdown of one's target.

Medical Impact - COVID Hospital Hesitancy

A new phenomenon, where there is a reduced inclination to go to the hospital, due to fears of contracting

COVID-19. Therefore, a new lack of effective healthcare delivery, particularly of (1) newly diagnosed conditions and (2) follow-up appointments of chronic conditions like diabetes, heart failure and COPD, has resulted in an increase in morbidity and mortality. Increased alcohol consumption, drug abuse epidemic and lower number of patients involved in smoking cessation has aggravated many patient's conditions. Psychological disorders have also emerged *de novo* or pre-existing conditions have exacerbated.

Social Determinants of Health

Although the capitalistic healthcare delivery system in the United States is nothing short of a tragedy, delivery and treatment only get worse during any sort natural calamity or man-made catastrophe, i.e., wars, famine and pandemics. There has been a disparity of healthcare availability and delivery in the US and around the globe. This imbalance has been further exacerbated by this current pandemic. The quality of treatment has been determined among cultural, racial and socioeconomic lines and status. This is even true internationally, even outside the realm of COVID. Cholera has been eradicated from affluent Western countries, but still wreaks havoc in the third world. Even within the most developed nations is there is a proverbial Fjord between the healthcare treatment of the wealthy and the poor. Those in the margins, like poor African communities in Louisiana, are hit particularly hard by the fight against the pandemic. A classic example is the plague of Marseille, where impoverished regions suffered and wealthy communities thrived.

Economic Implications

Whenever there is an outbreak or natural disaster, huge economic turbulence follows. Examples include floods, hurricanes, or a catastrophic pandemic. Not only are local economies impacted, but rather the world at large. Due to increasing globalization, we now find ourselves in a global village. Travel and business dealings across boundaries have made this pandemic even more difficult to control. Micro and macro economies have been negatively affected. For example, the lack of air and regular travel has put the airline and hospitality industries in a serious bind. Services suffer in hotels, restaurants, and conference centers. Therefore, good economic oversight, anticipation and preparation is needed to deal with any potential outbreak.

However, any given pandemic opens other opportunities as well, including the production of new medicine, PPE or more training or heftier requirements of new workforce. After the "storm" is over, medical and cross-vocational professionals should solidify damage control strategies for the future, to mitigate the negative effects of any future outbreaks or natural disasters. However, even with such strategies, it is always difficult to achieve pre pandemic results.

The term HRO or High Reliability Organizations was coined to depict models of healthcare and other sensitive industries like nuclear power plants, or aircraft nuclear carriers. These entities have to be reliable, because a slight mistake could cause a massive death toll, with a fallout for lasting decades. Another, strange phenomenon observed during the pandemic was the lack of a labor workforce. Partly, due to working from home, the risks of contracting COVID in the public, and also the realization that most low paying jobs are not worth the money for the risk.

Mitigation Strategies

Examined in the context of COVID-19 and other such pandemics, where the fallout of the disease causes several changes for the common man. Many strategies implemented by government officials are called mitigation strategies, because they try to dull the effect that the pandemic has had on society.

Shelter In Place-Stay Home-Lock down

A wartime phrase to let soldiers know that there is ordinance on their way, in the form of mortars or a nuclear attack. These orders are in place to try and minimize damage. A similar term is used in the field of epidemiology and public health during an epidemic or pandemic scenario where there is high transmissibility of the disease. The primary effect of a shelter in place order is to minimize the exposure of the infected person to the healthy population, and vice versa, to protect the healthy person from getting exposed to the diseased person. It also minimizes people on the street if the order functions properly. It can also be a form of government control, where rioters or looters (or Uncle Randy's Q-anon BBQ) are forced to vacate and stay at home.

Isolation Impact

A strict set of guidelines implemented after a contagious outbreak. This protocol is very strict, meaning that a very few medical personnel are allowed to enter a restricted or isolated area using rigid protocols and strict PPE requirements. A close record of all personnel entering and leaving the isolation wards is kept for contact tracing purposes, in the event that the site is responsible for further outbreak. Some countries and hospitals implemented these draconian measures to the letter. They had to balance the safety of the general population with the mental health of patients who sadly died in true isolation without seeing any family or friends during their last moments.

Social Distancing

With interaction being much higher in congested cities than somewhere like the suburbs, an order of 3-6 feet of healthy distancing plays a major role in minimizing personal contact. This is especially the case when the culprit is a highly contagious airborne illness like

COVID-19. This can also be the case in the event of a chemical attack, or some biochemical agent that can transfer from person to person. If the disease spreads through bodily secretion or air droplets, six feet orders will usually be implemented. Once a contagious disease is formally diagnosed, a more robust set of quarantine protocols may be required. The majority of outbreaks have deadly epicenters in overcrowded cities and countries with heavy urban areas, as air space is limited. Infected air particles are rife, and viral transmission and aerosolization through sneezing or coughing exacerbates an already deadly situation.

Spiritual Connection

Many have turned to religion and culture through the trying and isolating times of the pandemic. Psychological byproducts of stay-at-home orders should not be ignored. Connecting with one's family and loved ones, engaging with new hobbies, and perhaps even one's bond with a creator, can mitigate psychological decay. The state of mental health in the US has deteriorated further with the onset of this isolating virus, including an uptick in suicides. Mental health professionals and cross vocational studies should probe into how to prevent or mitigate this damage in the future.

Geographical Templating

Making testing and resources available at local levels, while enhancing hospital/ICU beds capacity by using various emergency hospital protocols. Having a pre-existing policy in place for testing and treating, will minimize the chaos during a "doomsday" scenario.

Population Health
The study of health in a group of people in certain geographic areas. Organizations like the WHO may embark on a specific study, like the study of diabetes or heart disease in a certain population, while trying to brainstorm strategies to diagnose and treat. This kind of study helps to drive measurable outcome data and metrics so practical approaches and calculated strategies can be implemented with far-ranging effectiveness. Childhood obesity is such an issue, with far ranging implications. Identification and mitigation strategies need to be put in place so future comorbid diseases such as diabetes and hypertension can be prevented on a larger scale.

Policy vs Politics
Local hospital, healthcare entities, whether public or private, need to be engaged in designing and implementing emergency policy and procedures according to public health agencies. Other regulatory agencies and authorities i.e., local CDC's and WHO should be actively involved in the design so they can be active partners during pandemics. Political figures need to be updated and involved as they are the voices and ears of the local populace.

Military Engagement

Military assets and personnel are later engaged when pandemics is out of proportion to preexisting civilian capabilities. The military can work independently, or in concert with local civil authorities to establish temporary hospitals or employ logistical help. During the Haitian earthquake, the military played an essential role in every aspect of humanitarian and healthcare help. Some of the military's services include:

- Command & Control
- Logistics
- Non-fighting Humanitarian Missions
- Corps of Engineers
- Medical Corps
- Chaplain Services

Quarantine

The legal definition of quarantine is a restriction on movement and can help thwart the spread of disease. This can be accomplished by imposing a self or obligatory mass quarantine. There are, however, medical and legal implications of imposing such a prohibitive and restrictive order.

Self-Quarantine

The reduction or elimination of outside contact from one's person. Commonly through isolating at home, this is the simplest and probably most effective strategy in prevention of the disease.

Obligatory Quarantine

A seemingly draconian measure, where isolation becomes mandatory for specified length of time. This term often refers to an out-patient measure. This order seems extreme in the scenario that a COVID patient is languishing alone in an ICU ward. They are not allowed to see their loved ones. Akin to the "solitary confinement" of a death row inmate, this form of isolation can result in detrimental outcomes. Mortality and morbidity of patients who are sick, but also psychologically compromised and isolated may expire quickly or have a lower success rate of treatment. There needs to be some sort of balance where the patient's mental health is taken into effect. For example, I was part of a study where ICU patients reduced the length of their ICU stays when walking was embedded into their treatment plans. Small changes in the mental health of the patient can go a long way to positively influence overall health and recovery time.

Behavioral Modification

UNLEARNING OLD BEHAVIORS

Humans are creatures of habit. Changing said patterns can be monumentally difficult. For the uninitiated, it can be very difficult to change a habit. The worst-case scenario could be total societal upheaval. Repeated behaviors and habits can find their roots in social and cultural norms, religious and even syncretic beliefs. These habits and social norms are shaped by preconceived notions and biases and are difficult to modify. Examples include shaking hands, hugging and grabbing coffee are day-to-day norms. Social distancing can disrupt these norms. Old habits die hard, and in our case, can spread disease.

LEARNING NEW BEHAVIOR
With a little bit of education and training, new behaviors can slowly be introduced. Learning new behavior and habits might be easier than getting rid of old habits. An order to wear a mask is a new behavior, rather than an example of subtracting an old habit.

Flattening the Curve
A statistical term that depicts the decrease of the rate of viral spread. Best visualized graphically, where the x axis displays the number of cases over time, in linear fashion. Usually, there is an initial spike followed by downtrend and plateau and ultimately flattening, which means the decrease of the rate of spread. Simple preventive measures like handwashing and social distancing can flatten the curve.

Measures taken during an epidemics

IDENTIFICATION
- Disease
- Pattern of spread
- Vectors
- Organisms i.e., virus, bacteria

PREVENTION
Disease specific measures, i.e., hand washing, social distancing.

MITIGATION
The key concept of mitigation is implementing measures to reduce the negative effects of an already ongoing crisis. Once an outbreak occurs, a set of "mitigation" measures can be set in place to help control the spread of disease. These steps could range from employing more resources to one particularly affected area, to the extension of a mask mandate in public and government places.

DAMAGE CONTROL
Damage control is the assessment of the negative impact of an event, with reduction or remediation measures that accompany the assessment. This can be done in either stages, or after the outbreak has died down. For example, damage control can be implemented once the organism has mutated,

therefore creating a wall between the old virus and the new form of the virus. This can be done for data gathering purposes and to help those in need. Damage control can be fine-tuned or large scale, ranging from the assessment of a suburb of New York, to addressing large scale societal grievances of working women.

Lessons Learned-Table Top-Hot Wash

Once these epidemics and pandemics have wreaked their havoc, the next step is to learn the lessons and help prepare for future outbreaks. This distinct lack of this preparation resulted in death and despair in the US and other developed nations. Perhaps our leaders should have heeded the calls when reports of a Wuhan virus started to float from the ether. The most common form of pandemic is usually respiratory, so it is not a difficult task to keep appropriate PPE and equipment such as ventilators at the ready.

Conspiracy Theories

Across the annals of history are rife with many misinformation campaigns. Nazi Germany turned a whole nation against its own people through such a maneuver. Wartime propaganda helped United States efforts across several wars, increasing enlistment and labor numbers across the board, even if demonizing an enemy that didn't deserve the flak. Conspiracy theories are a different animal. What started as fun conjecture over online message boards about aliens and secret government projects during World War 2, quickly degenerated into a sad lifestyle. Disaffected Americans believed that a mysterious insider in Washington was revealing a plot of total planned government control among other theories. The pandemic was not spared. These "theorists" deemed this pandemic the *"Plandemic,"* as a popular YouTube video by the same name made the rounds over Facebook, our favorite peddler of falsehoods. Conspiracy theories are harmful to the containment of this virus because a few are convincing the gullible many that the virus is a widespread tool of control implemented by the government to subtract personal rights. This could be furthest from the truth. The vaccine is not a tool of control, but a new technology designed to stop the virus most effectively in the host. Pandemic protocols are not in place to exert control over citizens but put in place to stop the virus. Even if we play devil's advocate, we see that releasing a virus into the world in order to control its citizens would be the worst thought-out plan in human history. Instead of more control, the government has, if anything, lost the control and support of its citizens because of the virus.

Telemedicine or Telehealth

Never before used in this scale, the telehealth paradigm of healthcare has gained such a widespread level of practicality and momentum through the pandemic. Some degree of telehealth did exist before COVID, especially in the field of psychiatry and pediatrics, and also between cities and small towns in remote areas of the United States. Tele-critical care or "E-ICU", or Electronic Intensive Care Units, did operate in most developed nations more so across the US than other countries. Social media tools and software, like Zoom, Skype and other proprietary programs have allowed physicians to treat even the most remote patients from all around the world. I know people who live in one state, and practice medicine in another due to the betterment of telehealth infrastructure. This paradigm is especially helpful in a COVID, high contagion setting.

Tele-education

Just like telemedicine, remote schooling and various tele-methodologies have also emerged during the pandemic. Even institutions of higher education have adopted remote methodologies, which are not limited to just Zoom. There are pluses and minuses to this delivery of education. The lack of social interaction and real world repercussions to student behavior has had a rather negative impact on the overall social and emotional development and health of young children. Kids of all ages lose the opportunity to be in a live setting. At home, not attending class, or scoring low on a test may not be regarded as such a detriment. Instead, students and young people must deal with daily existentialism, poor internet connection, and the lack of school lunches for those American children who rely on public schools for meals. It is the young people who are suffering the most and losing precious seconds of their childhood.

Regulatory Agencies-Governmental Organizations-NGO

Various governmental and non-governmental organizations who play an instrumental role during natural and man-made disasters. The roles of Red Cross-Red Crescent, Doctors without Borders and Peace Corp are evident and can be seen during these catastrophes. Some of the highest paid executives in the world work for nonprofits, and this is a very good thing. If there is greater incentive for NGO's and nonprofits to change the world for the better, it is possible that future pandemics or health care crises could be mitigated sooner.

State and County Regulated Agencies

Local agencies that offer governance and oversight to the delivery of healthcare services. These may include the state department of health, which is further subdivided into counties. These entities often work in conjunction with the federal as well operate based on their own unique population that it serves. The upsides are that these agencies know local needs and boundaries. Downsides may be the remoteness of the agency and county, and the lack of proper healthcare infrastructure and protocol.

FDA

This is a federal agency, which was founded by former President Teddy Roosevelt. From the FDA website: the "FDA is responsible for protecting the public health by ensuring the safety, efficacy, and security of human and veterinary drugs, biological products, and healthcare devices and equipment." It serves under the umbrella of the department of Health and Human Services (HHS). The positives to this agency are the widespread control and infrastructure it has to regulate healthcare objectives. Downsides could be that it cannot effectively take care of the needs for all Americans because of specific groups of people that need certain medical advice and treatment. For example, the FDA may craft a policy that helps white, urban and wealthy Americans that live in New York, more than it does poor, white Americans that live in Iowa.

HHS

The Department of Health and Human Services, is the federal department which oversees the overall administrative aspects of healthcare in the country. The FDA works under the direction of HHS.

CDC

The Center for Disease Control is the national public health agency of the USA. It is a federal agency which works under the auspices of HHS. This was founded in 1946, and is housed in Atlanta, Georgia. The primary mission of CDC is to safeguard the nations' health and safety from various diseases and threats that compromise the health and safety of the common American. The significance of CDC became widely known and accepted after the COVID-19 pandemic, which affected every citizen of the USA and the world at large. The CDC is the organization that has to analyze a lot of health data quickly and recommend to Americans the best course of action in a local and private setting. This is where mask mandates originate, as well as general healthcare policy and protocol in a pandemic setting.

FEMA

Federal Emergency Management Agency, is a subsidiary of the Department of Homeland Security (DHS), and deals with all emergencies and catastrophes caused by man-made or natural disasters such as hurricanes, tornados etc. Its role and failure became evident during hurricane Katrina. Its inception date was 1979, by President Jimmy Carter. FEMA is most broadly known for its boots-on-the-ground manpower and assistance.

OSHA

The Occupational Safety and Health Agency is a branch of the Department of Labor, which traces its roots during Nixon's era of 1971. This federal agency deals with the workplace environment, its safety and regulates and deploys various safety standards. It has the authority to inspect the workplace environment and can implement safety standards. It has far reaching goals to ensure the safety of workers.

NFPA
The National Fire Protection Association is an international non-for-profit organization that deals with protecting human life, preventing injury and providing safety from the hazards of fire.

JOINT COMMISSION
A non-for-profit organization that offers certification and accreditation to various healthcare facilities both governmental and private entities. It mostly deals with the safety and quality of healthcare delivery to the patients.

Zoonotic Disease

These diseases are transmitted from animals to humans. Zoonotic diseases can spread from animal to humans through direct contact, indirect contact, vector-borne, foodborne, or waterborne means. Some of the common diseases associated with animal or zoonotic transmission are listed below.

Cat Transmission
Toxoplasmosis: a zoonotic disease that can transfer from cats to humans. Toxo can infect pregnant women that touch the cat's litter box but can also be foodborne if poor hand hygiene is practiced. Cat transmission can cause serious complications including fetal anomalies and stillbirth.
Pasteurella: spread through aerosolized droplets when cats cough or through an infected cat bite as the Pasteurella species are natural inhabitants of the skin, digestive tract and oral cavity of cats.

Dogs

Pasteurella: spread through aerosolized droplets when a dog coughs or through an infected dog bite.

Rabies: the transmission of rabies from dog to human generally occurs after a bite from the infected animal when the infected saliva enters the human's system. However, people can get rabies if an open cut, wound, or abrasion is exposed to infected material from a rabid dog. Most dogs in the U.S are vaccinated. Raccoons and Bats are the leading causes of Rabies in the U.S.

Tick Borne Disease

Lyme disease: white tail deer is often the intermediate host.

Rocky Mountain Spotted Fever-RMSF

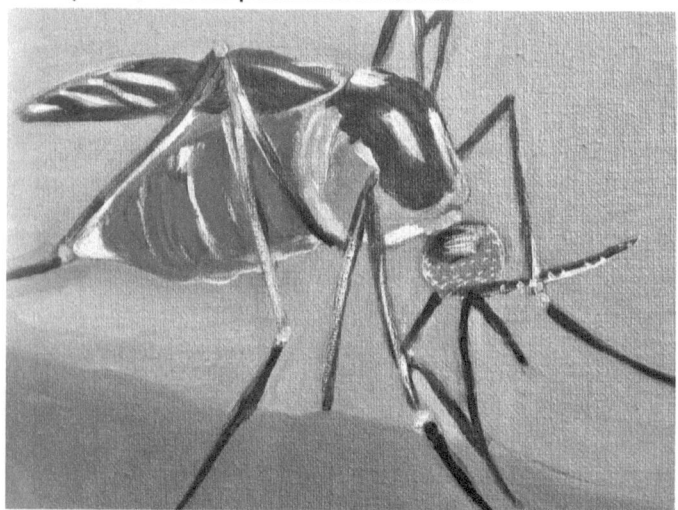

Khalida Anwar, MD

Mosquito-borne illnesses
Malaria
Dengue
West Nile
Eastern Equine Encephalitis
Zika
Chikungunya

These diseases are not endemic to the United States but are typically encountered in returning international travelers.

Avian-Birds
H1N1-Bird Flu
Psittacosis
Bird Fancier's Disease

Bovine-Cows
E coli
Ringworm disease
Salmonella
Mad Cow Disease-Prion Disease (Cruetz-Feld Jakob Disease).
Listeria-with infected and unpasteurized milk or cheese and its products.

Rodents
Hantavirus
Plague

Lassa Fever
Ebola

Bats (Flying Mammals)

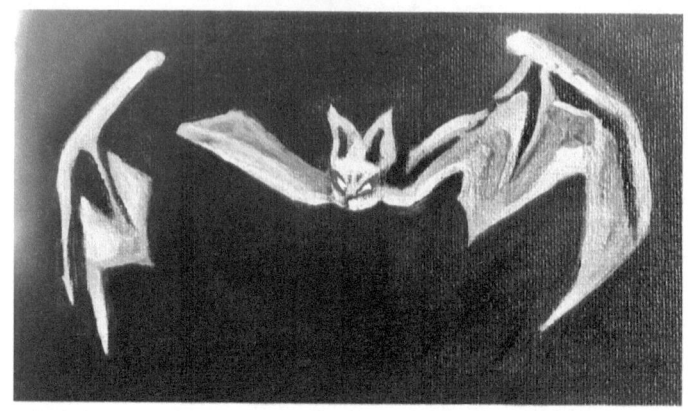

Khalida Anwar, MD

Corona
SARS
MERS
COVID-19
Ebola
Rabies

Porcine-Pigs
Swine Influenza A
H3 N2
H1N1
Campylobacter
Cryptosporidium

ZOONOTIC DISEASE

Leptospirosis
Rabies
Ringworm
Salmonella
Yersinia

Pangolins
COVID-19

PART II

CORONAVIRUS aka COVID-19 - SARS-CoV-2

Definition

The term COVID-19 is a novel type of the existent coronavirus disease, that spread in the year 2019. "Conventional Coronavirus" virus is a common human and animal pathogen, which has been present and has caused various upper respiratory diseases in the past, both in humans and animals. However, the epicenter of the "Novel Coronavirus" of 2019, was allegedly near Wuhan, a city in China. The breakout was reported to have occurred in December 2019. However, there has been a surge of *"Atypical Pneumonia"* even prior to the officially reported timeline of the COVID-19 cases, since October 2019, raising suspicions that the disease may have been infecting people before being officially declared by the CDC as a global emergency. Our ICU ward had many mysterious cases of long-lasting pneumonia and fatigue before COVID-19 made headlines, so it is possible that COVID was spreading long before.

Due to rapid spread, contagiousness and the mortality associated with this disease, it officially received the designation of pandemic in February 2019, by the World Health Organization (WHO). This disease has since been a major public health emergency and a consequential deadly global pandemic. The terms SARS-CoV-2 and COVID-19 will be used interchangeably through this text. Referred to as "China Virus," or "Wuhan virus," by right leaning political figures, and starting as *the coronavirus* in early news reports, the world has largely settled on the term "COVID."

SIGNS AND SYMPTOMS
"COVID SHOWS-HEAD TO TOES"

CONSTITUTIONAL

New onset of fever, chills, myalgia and generalized malaise, the loss of taste and smell along with specific systemic manifestations. The infected person does not have to have all the symptoms to be suspected for COVID infection as one set of symptoms may suffice. Some patients may be asymptomatic and may not have any symptoms, at least initially.

Respiratory Symptoms
- Cough
- Shortness of breath
- Hypoxia (mostly asymptomatic) i.e., *Happy Hypoxia or Silent Hypoxia*
- Chest pain-pleuritic in nature
- Upper or Lower Respiratory Tract Infections
- Respiratory Failure - which may require any supplemental oxygenation or ventilatory support, non-invasive positive pressure ventilation or mechanical ventilation

Gastrointestinal
- Nausea, vomiting, diarrhea, abdominal pain
- Loss of taste and smell
- COVID-19 tongue
- Hepatopathy-abnormal liver enzymes

Hematological System
- Coagulopathy-mostly procoagulant in nature
- Disseminated Intravascular Coagulation (DIC)
- Elevated Fibrinogen
- Elevated D-Dimer
- Thrombocytosis or Thrombocytopenia
- Deep Venous Thrombosis, DVT (Leg Clots)
- Pulmonary Embolism, PE (Lung Clots)

Central Nervous System
- Confusion and forgetfulness, "COVID FOG"

- Encephalopathy-delirium to memory deficits
- Stroke-mostly ischemic or thrombotic in nature

CARDIOVASCULAR SYSTEM
- Chest pain
- Acute Coronary Syndrome, MI, myocarditis, epicarditis
- Limb vascular ischemia
- Arrhythmias-abnormal heart rhythm

MUSCULOSKELETAL SYSTEM
- Peripheral nerve involvement causing loss of taste and smell
- Diaphragmatic muscle involvement causing fibrosis and shortness of breath

DERMATOLOGICAL/SKIN ISSUES
- Kawasaki Disease "pediatric population"
- Morbilliform Rash
- Urticarial Rash
- *"COVID TOES"* a peculiar rash on toes, contracted during pedicure
- Contact Rash "PPE Rash" has been reported in healthcare workers across the board. This results either from mere friction or abrasions vs allergic manifestation.
- Cessation of immune-modulating drugs for skin condition-Initially there was a fear of

contracting COVID-19 infection due to these drugs, however, this proved to be unsubstantiated and the one the treatment was resumed, there were no such sequelae noted. As a result, initial withholding of these meds resulted in exacerbation of the rash.

Epidemiology

Travel history is of less importance due to the global reach of the pandemic. Travel restrictions are still necessary to ascertain contact in the higher cluster area or community contact with a person with known or suspected COVID-19. This is useful for contact tracing and surveillance of various strains. Advanced age and underlying medical conditions show worsening disease. Case fatality rate is 2-5% on average and goes up to 15% in the older age group.

Transmission:

Zoonotic Transmission

Contact with infected animals; bats are suspected as vectors in this particular case. There have been reports of minks as potential vectors of the disease as well, leading to a significant culling of certain mink populations.

Human-Human

The most prominent mode of transmission.

Large Particles >5 microns
- Droplet
- Travels long distance more than 6 feet
- Cough
- Sneezing
- May cause upper respiratory symptoms, tracheitis and bronchitis

Small Particles < 2.5 microns
- Remain airborne for a long time
- Travels short distances 6 feet or less
- Spread by talking, laughing
- Can cause severe lung infection, i.e., pneumonia as has the ability to penetrate deeper into the lungs

Contact
- Touching an infected person
- Contact with mucous membrane
- Contact with infected surface

Fecal
- Less likely-even though, virus sheds in feces

Sexual Transmission
There were some case reports where the virus was found in the seminal fluid of the infected males. Hence, if becomes an effective mode of transmission, may render SARS CoV-2 as a Sexually Transmitted Disease (STD).

Incubation Period:
- 14 days is suggested; hence the length of quarantine should last at least that long.
- 7-day quarantine has been suggested by CDC in certain asymptomatic cases.

Course of Illness:
Varies from person to person, depending on host defenses response, and underlying immunogenic response in addition to co-morbid conditions.

Asymptomatic Carriers
A person with intact immunity may get colonized and not infected with the disease, but can shed virus and infect other people, which was the most common occurrence around the world. Younger age groups were the most common carriers since they were mostly asymptomatic despite having continued social interaction. leading to more public adventuring. This disseminated the virus across multiple locales and also spreading symptomatic infection at home, if they were cohabitating with elderly.

Non-life-threatening Disease: >80%
- Flu like symptoms
- Fever
- Fatigue
- Anosmia and dysgeusia

- Lower respiratory symptoms
  - Cough-dry
  - Shortness of breath
  - Congestion
- Gastrointestinal symptoms
  - Nausea-Vomiting
  - Diarrhea

Critical Illness-Life Threatening Illness

Worsening symptoms requiring ER visit or hospitalization.

Admission to ICU with:

ACUTE RESPIRATORY FAILURE
- Hypoxic respiratory failure-most common type
- Hypercarbic respiratory failure

PNEUMONIA
- COVID-19 Pneumonia
- Post Viral Pneumonia
- Superimposed bacterial Pneumonia

ARDS - ACUTE RESPIRATORY DISTRESS SYNDROME
- Bilateral ground glass opacities
- P/F (pO2 divided by the Fio2) ratio <300 -normal more than 300

THE NEW PANDEMIC

- Age > 65 years - more common in higher age bracket
- Diabetes Mellitus
- Hypertension
- Smokers tend to have worsening disease and respiratory failure
- Obesity

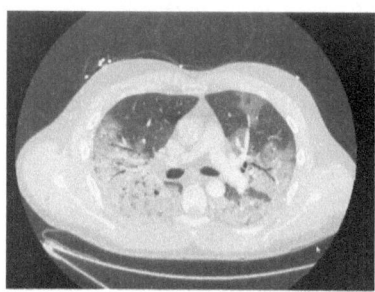 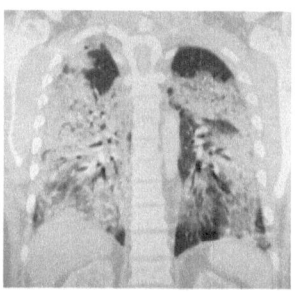

CT scan of COVID-19 pneumonia and ARDS (white area-pneumonia is disease and black-air is normal)

MULTI-ORGAN FAILURE

SEPTIC SHOCK, APPROXIMATELY 5.0%
- Requiring vasopressor support for hemodynamic support

CNS
- CVA-Stroke-thrombotic
- Encephalitis/encephalopathy
- Locked in syndrome

Cardiovascular
- Myocardial Infarction (MI)
- Myocarditis
- Pericarditis
- Ventricular wall rupture

Coagulopathies
- Elevated D-Dimer
- Deep Venous Thrombosis - DVT
- Pulmonary Embolism
- DIC pattern - Disseminated Intravascular Coagulation

Dermatological
- Skin Rash-generalized
- "COVID Toes"-a peculiar rash on the feet and digits

Cytokines Storm
Elevated inflammatory markers or cytokines, IL-6 and others:
- CRP - C Reactive Proteins
- LDH - Lactic Dehydrogenase
- Ferritin
- D-Dimer
- Erythrocyte Sedimentation Rate -ESR or Sed Rate

Diagnosis

Diagnosis is based on a myriad of signs and symptoms. It can vary from asymptomatic carrier to manifestation of critical illness. Initially, it was associated with travel to high-risk areas, i.e., Wuhan, China, Italy or New York. Later, due to widespread community related transmission, it became a community spread disease and now is a major pandemic.

Laboratory tests

The first question is to decipher why a particular test is performed, when it is performed, and what kind of test is best performed. There are "Four Why's" included in this analysis that one needs to ask, before a test becomes reliable and results valid.

The following flow diagram depicts this series of questioning clearly, and if one follows the algorithm, they can see if it is the desired and anticipated rationale for performing a specific test. This is a generic conceptualization and methodology of performing any test. Also, whenever a test is performed there should be an intention to treat it.

CORONAVIRUS AKA COVID-19 - SARS-COV-2

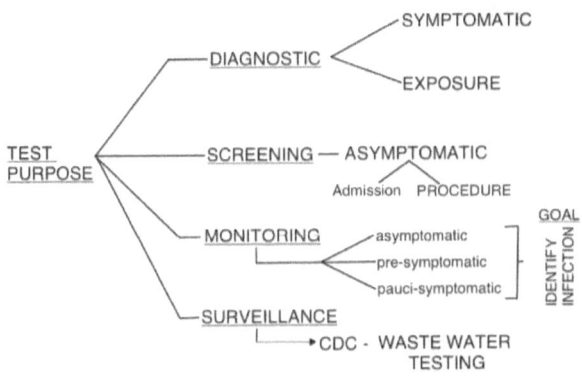

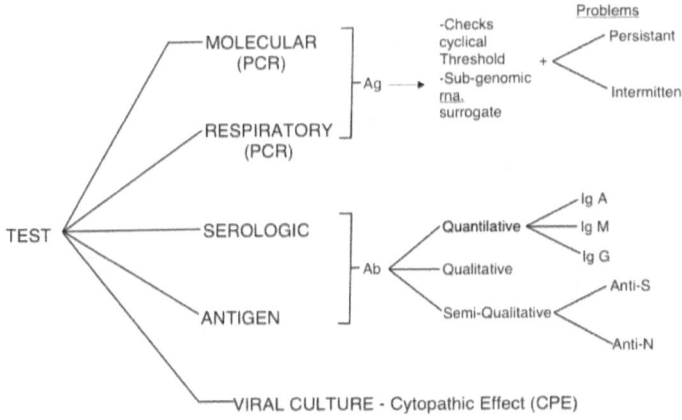

TESTS for the COVID-19 infection
- Rapid Test (Antigen or PCR testing)
- Nasopharyngeal swab or sputum sample to test for Reverse Transcriptase Polymerase Chain Reaction (RT PCR)

- FLUVID (tests SARS-CoV-2-Flu and RSV viruses)
- Bronchoscopy specimens can also be obtained if unable to get specimens conventionally
- CBC- look at the differential white blood cell count - Lymphopenia
- Elevated D Dimer
- Elevated Lactic Dehydrogenase - nLDH
- Elevated ferritin
- Elevated acute phase reactants i.e., CRP, ESR
- Procalcitonin (biological marker of bacterial infection)-often normal
- Abnormal liver function, i.e., AST and ALT

Radiological Findings
Chest X-Ray
  Bilateral infiltrates

CT Chest
  Bilateral infiltrates, with associated manifestations of:
  - Ground glass rounded appearance
  - Lower lobe predominance, around peripheral parenchyma
  - Thickened pleura
  - Lymphadenopathy

CORONAVIRUS AKA COVID-19 - SARS-COV-2

Treatment Regimen

This can include generalized measures, symptomatic management and pharmacological interventions

Generalized Measures

Mild disease
- Home Care on out-patient basis
- Strict quarantine 7-14 days
- Supportive care, hydration, Over the Counter - OTC meds acetaminophen as needed
- Tele-medicine assistance

Moderate-Critical Disease:
- Immediate isolation in single room infirmary units, if available.
- Preferably a negative isolation room with HEPA filtration system, which became very challenging due to non-availability, therefore regular rooms were utilized for most hospital admissions.
- Infection control measures should be instituted including PPE.
- Use *anteroom* prior to entering the negative pressure room, if available.
- Strict hand washing or alcohol-based cleaning agents.
- Using sign-in sheets for healthcare personnel entering, done initially for

contact tracing and minimizing the time and duration of exposure in a particular shift, later this practice was discontinued since there was a surge of cases.
- Close monitoring of vital signs, including oximetry.

Symptomatic treatment

Supplemental oxygen
- To keep the Oxygen saturation by pulse oximetry i.e., "Spo2" >90%, in an otherwise healthy individual, since they suffer from "Happy Hypoxia" as they don't exhibit many hypoxic symptoms.
- Over The Counter "OTC" meds for symptomatic relief of fever, i.e., acetaminophen.

Non-Invasive Positive Pressure Ventilation (NIPPV)
- To keep Spo2 >90%, along with ventilatory support via CPAP, BiPAP, AVAPS.

Ventilatory Support
- Early intubation for acute hypoxic respiratory failure was recommended

initially, but later proved to be more detrimental as the mortality increased in the intubated patients.
- Low Tidal Volume Strategy was implemented i.e., 6-8 cc/kg ideal body weight-if and when the patient is intubated.
- Conservative fluid management per ARDS protocol i.e., keep Central Venous Pressure CVP <6, if not requiring vasopressors.
- Avoidance of Non-Invasive Positive Pressure ventilatory devices NIPPV, i.e., BiPAP, AVAPS, CPAP, HFNO etc. as these are believed to result in aerosolization of viral inoculum and are associated with higher mortality.
- Minimizing delivery of nebulization medication. However, still used due to paucity of the quality data which provides significant pros and cons of use of this treatment modality.
- Nitric Oxide as an adjunct to conventional high Fio2 when refractory hypoxemia sets in and (Positive End Expiratory Pressure) PEEP can't be escalated beyond a certain threshold.

Prone Position Ventilation

Recommended in both non-intubated "awake proning" or "self proning" and intubated patients particularly in severe ARDS P/F ratio <150 i.e., "arterial oxygen saturation Sao2 divided by fractionated oxygen provided by Fio2."

Bronchoscopy

Bronchoscopy is a recommended procedure for the mucus clearance and sample collection. However, it was discouraged initially, as there was an increased potential for aerosolization of the viral inoculum in the air. In the later phase of endemics, it became inevitable in some cases, where an ET tube would clog up, and either the Endotracheal Tube "ET" tube had to be changed with the tube exchanger or multiple bronchoscopies were performed to clean the airways. Hence, bronchoscopies help improve ventilation and oxygenation. Several patients, especially those who tested positive for PPD or were on Tocilizumab, were tested for Acid Fast Bacilli "AFB" organism which causes TB.

VACCINES

There is only one FDA approved vaccine (Pfizer) currently available:

Pfizer (Comirnaty)
(two shots 21 days apart)   95% safe and effective
Moderna
(two shots 28 days apart)
                               95% safe and effective
Johnson & Johnson
(single dose) - can be stored in fridge temp 40-degree F
Sinopharm
BIBP-CorV
(China) (two shots 30 days apart)-Inactivated Virus

There are a few others in the vaccination repertoire and are expected in the coming weeks and months. There are yet a few others in the pipeline, with various timelines and efficacies and ease of administration. There were some side effects reported due to vaccines *per se*, however, not enough to mandate "black label warning."

PHARMACOLOGICAL INTERVENTION - TRIED/TESTED

Off Label Use Products:

- Chloroquine and Hydroxychloroquine (No longer has Emergency use authorization or EUA)

In vitro success-emergent received FDA approval; 400 mg, PO BID for 2 days and then 200 BID for 5 days (max 14 days). There are reported cardiac arrhythmias associated with the use, without significant benefits; therefore, emergency approval was reversed, and its widespread use was discontinued worldwide. This intervention had proven to be more of a political stunt rather than a product of pure scientific data analysis.
- Lopinavir-ritonavir (did not get much steam and wasn't used).
- Oseltamivir-Tamiflu (although proven to be effective for the flu virus wasn't not widely used during the COVID-19 epidemic).
- Discontinuing ACE-I/ARB (altered ACE levels were suspected in the etiology of this disease, hence resulting in stopping the ACE-I/ARBs. However, further studies refuted this physiologic and pharmacologic concern. Therefore, a normal approach in initiating and discontinuing of this pharmacologic intervention was recommended as an anti-hypertensive medication, which was independent of presence of COVID-19 infection.
- Interferon (wasn't used).
- Conventional Antibiotics-Azithromycin-Rocephin-quinolones

    These antimicrobials were used routinely and empirically on literally every patient who was admitted to the hospital with COVID-19 infection. Even though the drug didn't have any specific indication for the treatment of COVID-19, it was given to cover community-acquired elements especially in the setting of elevated procalcitonin.

- Vit-C (CITRUS-ALI TRIAL)
  Vit-C alone or in combination did not offer much of benefit, albeit it was widely used initially during the COVID-19 surge.
- Convalescent Serum or plasma obtained from patients who recovered from COVID-19 infection had antibodies against the virus. This plasma was harvested from those patients and transfused to newly infected COVID-19 patients to provide passive titers of neutralizing antibodies which can render passive immunity. So far, this strategy has not been proven to be a major clinical modifier, but some NEJM studies published in January 2021, reported that transfusion of plasma with higher antibodies in patients not on mechanical ventilation may be associated with a lower risk of death. It has been given EAU by the DEA.
- Melatonin (initially used and later became less favorable).
- Pepcid did not prove to confer any additional benefits, therefore was later discontinued.

- Zinc (supplement, which gained some momentum, but later did not prove to be of significant benefit. Its use is being considered for post-exposure prophylaxis on an out-patient basis. Various studies done across the globe in India and Argentina failed to show survival benefits. However, these clinical trials are still early and lack certain characteristics.
- Ivermectin
  This medication has been widely used in the field of veterinary medicine and across the world especially in the developing countries for the treatment of parasitic worms/helminthic infection i.e., body lice or worm infestation including pinworm, hookworms. It was used in some parts of the world and initial studies showed some benefits. However, it did not get much steam in the Western World because of the lack of benefits in COVID-19 treatment. Ivermectin was not approved by the FDA for its use even with Emergency Use Authorization, "EUA." The JAMA article "Effects of Ivermectin on Time to Resolution of Symptoms Among Adults with Mild COVID-19 Trial," published March 2021 did not improve the time to resolution. I have seen many patients who refuse to take the vaccine and traditional COVID prevention methods, and demand ivermectin because of a successful

conspiracy theory touting ivermectin as more effective than the mRNA vaccines. One wonders whether the opposite would be true if indeed Ivermectin were indeed the most effective COVID treatment.

FDA APPROVED MEDICATIONS
- Tocilizumab-anti-IL-6 (*REMAP-CAP* and *RECOVERY-Tocilizumab* Trials).
- Remdesivir-*Veklury* (broad-spectrum antiviral-nucleotide prodrug of adenosine analog).
- Bamlanivimab-Etesevimab (a monoclonal antibody is recommended along with Remdesivir).
- Steroids-Dexamethasone 6 mg daily or BID as an adjunct to the COVID regimen, shown to reduce mortality in the RECOVERY Trial.
- Thromboprophylaxis vs treatment - Lovenox-heparin-NOACS-*tPA*.

INSPIRATION trial- JAMA shows standard dose Enoxaparin 40 mg vs intermediated dose of 1 mg/kg divided twice daily, did not show non-inferiority of the standard dose and the bleeding complications were much higher than with an intermediate dose. There were also much higher reports of thrombocytopenia with an intermediate dose and no difference in the formation of the clot or serious outcome, therefore a standard dose is suggested.

Medications to Avoid
- NSAIDS-Not a strong recommendation.

Pulmonary Vasodilators
- Nitric Oxide
- Prostacyclin
- Flolan-may be limited as a nebulized or IV

ECMO
Veno-venous V-V ECMO can be used in patients with refractory hypoxemia, however the initial outcomes in ARDS and refractory hypoxemia were not very promising. This strategy proved to be efficacious and lifesaving during the last epidemic of H1N1. There has been a stark contrast between COVID-19 and H1N1, where much younger age group patients were afflicted with this disease and were especially helpful in saving the lives of pregnant females.

Discharging patients from the hospital
Disease symptoms are declared resolved when there are at least two negative laboratory samples, but due to the surges, not enough testing supplies were available, at least initially. Therefore, this practice was discontinued.

Patients should be advised to self-quarantine for 2 weeks even after a negative test. Later, this time recommendation was decreased to 7-10 days.

COVID-19 Clinical Course

80% mild symptoms,
14% severe symptoms requiring hospitalization,
5% critical care-ICU.

2-14 days after exposure
On day 5 patients present with "flu like" symptoms, i.e., fever, headache, dry cough, malaise, myalgias, nausea, abdominal discomfort with some diarrhea, loss of smell, anorexia, and fatigue.

Day 5 of symptoms
Dyspnea or cough
Usually bilateral viral pneumonia, however even unilateral pneumonia may be indicative of the disease. CT chest shows bilateral, peripheral lower lobe ground glass opacities.

Day 10
Cytokine surge leads to acute ARDS, which results in capillary leak syndrome resulting in difficulty ventilating and oxygenating.

Rapid onset of multiorgan failure ensues resulting in respiratory, cardiac and renal failure. Patient presentation is varied since this is such a dynamic disease. The majority of patients are coming in quite hypoxic without a subjective feeling of shortness of breath. Other presentations can vary from patient to patient and may present with encephalopathy, renal failure from dehydration, DKA, especially with exacerbation of preexisting underlying comorbid conditions.

Cardiac involvement occurs in about 15% of patients. These cardiac manifestations may vary from myocarditis, pericarditis, new onset CHF and new onset atrial fibrillation. For both COVID or Non-COVID-19 STEMIs are getting tPA in the ED and rescue PCI at 60 minutes only if tPA fails.

Diagnostic

Radiology

Initial radiologic testing by CXR shows bilateral pneumonia, but it often starts in the RLL, so bilateral on CXR is not required. The hypoxia is out of proportion to the findings on the CXR. Lung's auscultation may not be abnormal, therefore, rely on other clinical indicators such as tachypnea or hypoxia.

Labs

Once the patient meets the criteria for admission to the hospital, routine labs and diagnostic studies may be indicated, however, don't wait for COVID testing to treat the patient. The following are some of the studies, indicative of disease:

Leukopenia

Lymphopenia

Thrombocytopenia or thrombocytosis.

Procalcitonin, which is a sign of bacterial infection, is often normal.

CRP and Ferritin (acute phase reactants) are elevated most often.

CPK, D-Dimer, LDH, Alk Phos/AST/ALT are commonly elevated since they are acute phase reactants.

Therefore, interpret D-Dimer, if ordered with abundance of precautions as treading towards the wrong pathway i.e., pursuit of DVT/PE can result in further imaging with contrast studies, CT PE rendering these often-dehydrated patients to loads of contrast further deteriorating kidney function and resulting in acute kidney failure.

A ratio of absolute neutrophil count to absolute lymphocyte counts greater than 3.5 could be a poor prognostic sign.

An elevated Interleukin-6 (IL6) is a proinflammatory cytokine that can be an indicator of their cytokine surge, however, its utility as a diagnostic test is limited due to lack of rapid turnaround time. Therefore, it is suggested that we should refrain from testing it. However, if the patient is in dire straits and critical, and other modalities have failed anti-IL 6, Tocilizumab infusion can be considered as a compassionate use. Thrombocytopenia and elevated LFTs can be poor prognostic signs.

Disposition or Discharge from the hospital or ER

Discharge with oxygen if the patient is comfortable and oxygenating above 92% on the nasal cannula.

Advise patients to acquire a pulse oximeter, so they can check their oxygen levels, while at home.

Treatment

Supportive for mild symptoms.

86% of COVID-19 patients that go on ventilatory support may die as a sequela of the disease or its complications. Patients can be successfully extubated as soon as they meet the extubation criteria, which should be assessed daily.

Plaquenil has weak ACE2 receptor blockade, which was considered beneficial; however, there was QT prolongation and liver toxicity and lack of efficacy, therefore it was discontinued and EUA was revoked.

Azithromycin, in doses of 500 mg once daily IV or PO for 5-10 days.

Judicious use of resuscitation fluids should be considered as volume overload can hasten respiratory decompensation (which was initially reported as beneficial in the ARDSNET trial). Fluid overload status may result in intubation and mechanical ventilation as non-invasive modalities of ventilation were initially discouraged to mitigate the spread of virus through aerosolized routes. However, in case of DKA and renal failure and dehydration, justified use of fluids may be required.

"Proning" ventilated patients has proven oxygenation benefits. If the prone bed is available, it should be used; otherwise, regular beds with 16 hours of proning and every two-hour neck turn should be implemented. Even "self proning" or "awake proning" the ones on the nasal cannula can be helpful to move the fluid around lungs, and redirect the oxygen to less ventilated areas, in awake, alert and cooperative patients.

Vent settings- Usual ARDSNet protocol, low tidal volume ventilatory strategy, permissive hypercapnia, etc. except for PEEP of 5 will not do. Start at 14 and you may go up to 25 if needed.

Intubate late. Non-invasive modalities of ventilation and oxygenation and ventilation should be highly encouraged, these include BiPAP, CPAP, AVAPS. These methods of oxygenation and ventilatory support may result in significant exposure risk with high levels of aerosolized virus. Even after a cough or sneeze this virus can be aerosolized for up to 3 hours, or longer.

All nebulizer treatments should be used with caution and switched to Metered Dose Inhalers (MDI), whenever possible. Use MDI. you can give 8-10 puffs at one time of an albuterol MDI. If you must give a nebulizer, it is preferred to be in a negative pressure room and instruct the patient on how to start it after you leave the room, if possible.

NSAIDS use is discouraged; instead, acetaminophen should be utilized.

Steroid use early in the course of the illness was also not recommended, however, due to cytokine surge and pro-inflammatory cytokine storm, IV or oral steroids have shown significant benefit in reducing the detrimental effects of the inflammation earlier in the course of the disease process.

Anti-IL6 antibody Tocilizumab has been used in some patients; however, it is not only cost prohibitive but also lacks any clear evidence of clinical efficacy at this juncture. Therefore, the risks versus benefits ratio should be weighed before costly therapies.

SEDATION IN THE ICU
Versed, Fentanyl, Propofol, Precedex, Ketamine, Ativan, Phenobarbital and neuromuscular blocking agents i.e., Nimbex.

PPE
Strict respiratory, contact and droplet precautions need to be exercised, even when fully vaccinated.

NEGATIVE PRESSURE ROOMS
It is preferable to house COVID patients in a negative pressure room, attached to Anteroom. However, this was not a widespread practice due to the paucity of the negative pressure rooms and the overwhelming number of patients that crowded the healthcare system.

COVID-19 MILITARY TRIAGE RESPONSE
HEALTH LEVELS
The majority of the military installations resorted to uniform and standard measures.

No Symptoms-Asymptomatic Carriers
- Represent majority of the cases
- Temperature under 100 F
- No cough, sore throat, body aches, or shortness of breath

Action:
- Self-Observation/quarters/quarantine for two weeks
- RTD (Return to Duty) two weeks of quarantine
- If exposed follow guidelines from COVID-19 exposure flow chart

Mild Symptoms
- Temperature over 100 F
- New mild cough or sore throat
- New mild shortness of breath
- New body aches
- No other new symptoms

Action:
- Self-Monitoring or self-observation
- Monitors for worsening symptoms
- Isolate service member
- Not monitored by medical personnel
- Contact Lead at the MTF (Military Treatment Facility)

Moderate Symptoms
- Temperature over 100 F
- Shortness of breath
- Cough
- SpO2 greater than or equal to 94%
- Respiratory rate between 10 and 26 per minute

Action:
- Medic Monitoring
- Isolate and monitor by medical personnel in isolation

Severe Symptoms
- Shortness of breath or respiratory distress
- Persistent chest pain or chest pressure
- New onset of confusion or altered mental status
- Blushed or bluish lips or face
- Oxygen saturation or SpO2 under 94%
- Respiratory rate over 26 under 10 per minute

Action:
- Evacuation to Higher Echelon, higher level of care
- Call 911 to transport them to a hospital and update the Lead Medical Officer

COMPLICATIONS

Since, we have entered into the chronic phase of the disease, we are learning something new every day, including diagnosis, treatment, vaccination and its impact on the population at large. Some observations of long COVID follow.

POST COVID-19 SYNDROME
Aka "Long Haul COVID"
Long COVID-19 Syndrome
There are a unique set of systemic manifestations that may occur, even after the patient has been infected, symptomatic or asymptomatic, treated or untreated a while back. When tested they are negative on PCR and antibodies are present. This constellation of signs and symptoms is termed "Long COVID-19 syndrome" or patients have called themselves as "Long Haulers."

The manifestations of long COVID are quite similar to what was observed post MERS and SARS, which are both coronavirus diseases. This includes fatigue months after negative tests, as well as lingering loss of taste, smell and inability to concentrate.

POST-VIRAL PNEUMONIA
Often bacterial or fungal in immunocompromised patients, requiring a prolonged course of antibiotics and antifungal agents.
- Cough
- Dyspnea
- Chest pain

POST COVID CHRONIC HYPOXIC RESPIRATORY FAILURE
Often requiring supplemental oxygen.
Some patients may need Noninvasive Positive Pressure Ventilation-NIPPV, BiPAP, AVAPS.

Post COVID Pulmonary Fibrosis
Interstitial Lung Disease-ILD-not yet clearly proven, but there appears to be long term sequelae of the COVID-19 infection that necessitates oxygen requirement. Future studies, including imaging and PFTs will provide additional evidence and significance to that effect.

Post COVID Cardiac Manifestation
- Chest Pain
- Arrhythmias
- Palpitations

Post COVID Thromboembolism
- PE
- DVT

Post COVID Neurological Issues
- Encephalopathy
- Cognitive disturbances or "Brain Fog"
- Strokes
- Seizures
- Headaches
- Anxiety - depression
- Circadian and other sleep disorders

Post COVID Dermatological Problems
- COVID-19 toes
- Hair Loss

Post COVID Generalized Problems
- Generalized fatigue
- Muscular weakness
- Joint and muscle pain
- Decline in overall quality of life

Post COVID Renal Problems
- Acute Kidney Injury or AKI
- Acute on Chronic Renal Failure - CRF

Post COVID worsening of underlying chronic medical conditions

These manifestations could be secondary to either worsening due to COVID-19 related pathogenesis or inability to seek help during pandemics which resulted in non-compliance with the treatment regimen. Some examples are:
- DM-erratic glycemic index and poor to control diabetes
- Thyroid diseases
- Cardiac condition-CHF

Post ICU syndrome (PICS)

A close cousin of Post-Traumatic Stress Syndrome (PTSD) consisting of physical, mental and emotional symptomatology that occurs and may persist days to months after a patient is treated and discharged from the intensive care unit. Even though its presence is well known, its presentation is quite subtle and only recently recognized in COVID-19 patients. This phenomenon of PICS is becoming more profound after the COVID-19 epidemic, which has resulted in more ICU days of care and prolonged illness.

COVID Related Transmission and Mortality in a Double Lung Transplant Recipient

The first case report in Michigan has been reported and presented of death in a transplant recipient. A lung transplant donor died of non-COVID-19 related causes and was tested negative before lungs were harvested. However, once transplanted with double lungs, the recipient was infected with COVID-19 and died of complications. Even the surgeon who harvested the lungs got infected, however later recovered.

Airborne SARS-CoV-2

Recent studies, published in Respiratory Research, showed characterization of hospital airborne SARS-CoV-2. The research concluded that even though the majority of spread and transmission of COVID-19 is attributed to the large particle >10 micron in droplet transmission. Airborne particles <2.5 microns did not get much steam. Therefore, only six feet and close contact was discouraged. However, a small particulate size was identified in the local hospital in Boston and showed its ability to remain airborne for a protracted period of time. There was less presence of the small airborne particles in the COVID-19 wards, or where strict guidelines of proper attire and PPE were followed. The small particle content was much higher in the non-COVID-19 ward or where there was more staff congregation and less use of PPE. This study indicates that small airborne particles may play a major role in the transmission of the airborne respiratory diseases and use of mitigating and preventive strategies i.e., negative pressure room and proper use of the PPE reduces such transmission.

Exercise Induced Hypoxia in post COVID-19 asymptomatic aviators has been observed when challenged with submaximal exercise testing on a treadmill (Bruce Protocol).

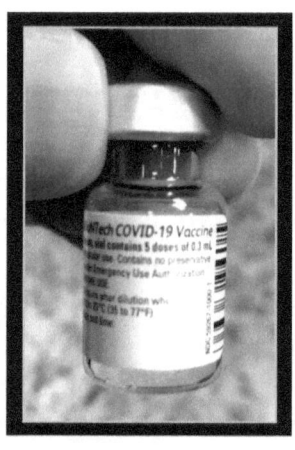

COVID vaccine - December 2020

Vaccine Breakthrough Infections

A breakthrough infection is a new infection in a fully vaccinated patients after four weeks of receiving the second dose. This is due to the rapidly emerging resistant strains. Even though the majority of the approved and studied vaccines show more than 80% immunity to even the highly resistant and emerging strains, mainly Delta as of the writing of this book. t Breakthrough infections are a known phenomenon that can occur after any type of vaccination. In some individuals, the vaccine confers "incomplete immunity," hence these people get infected besides optimal doses of vaccination. A similar pattern is being recognized in fully vaccinated patients. Even though the three currently available viruses confer 94% protection against severe COVID infection and death, this protection carries over about 80% protection against the new strain. Since the vaccine is not 100% effective against the virus, "mask wearing and continued social distancing and hand washing still need to continue, ideally until 80-90% of the global population gets vaccinated. This concept is known as herd immunity. Breakthrough infections are usually mild but severe cases and mortality have also been reported.

Another potentially beneficial strategy is the administration of booster vaccine doses, to reactivate memory cells at frequent intervals. The shingles vaccine is an example of the booster vaccine. *Lambda* variants have since emerged, causing outbreaks mostly in states with the lowest vaccination rate. The current Delta strain is thriving in the unvaccinated.

Covid-19 Vaccine Side Effects

Local

Pain and redness at the infection site

Systemic

Fever, chills, malaise, myalgias
Effects due to clotting enhancement of the clotting cascade DVT - Deep Venous Thrombosis (venous clots in extremities)
PE - Pulmonary Embolism (clot in the lungs)
CVA - Cerebral Vascular Accident or Stroke

Symptomatic Acute Myocarditis-adolescent patients

Clinical Presentation

Fever

Diagnosis

Elevated cardiac enzymes, troponins

> MRI with Gadolinium showed changes consistent with myocarditis

Treatment:

> NSAIDS - Non-Steroidal Anti-inflammatory Drugs such as Ibuprofen

IVIG- Intravenous Immunoglobulins) in selected cases

EFFICACY OF VACCINES OF THE "LONG HAULERS" OR LONG COVID SYNDROME

Recent post marketing analysis of the COVID=-19 vaccine has proven its efficacy in reducing the symptom complex of fatigue, muscle and "brain fog" even in patients with Long Covid Syndrome. Notably, Moderna was >30% effective in reduction of those symptoms, closely followed by Pfizer at 25%. J&J did not seem to offer that additional benefit, at least by evidence that has emerged so far.

ROLE OF OTHER VIRAL INFECTIONS ON SARS-C0V-2

Recent study, published in *The Journal of Infectious Disease*, March 23, 2021, reports that Human Rhinovirus Replication within Respiratory Epithelium Blocks SARS CoV-2 replication. This virus to virus interaction somehow offers a protective role, by retarding growth and spread of COVID-19 infection. There is a hypothetical competitive advantage of other viruses over SARS CoV-2. However, further studies will elucidate potential implications of population health and spread of this pandemic.

Decompensated Syndrome

Although not a scientific term, an effective expression underlying the gross neglect of other underlying medical conditions such as heart and kidney failure. This was initially due to the unavailability of outpatient clinics, personnel and later due to the availability of tele-health. Lack of regular and routine testing was not performed, therefore pre-existing medical conditions worsened.

This trend also affected cancers and other medical conditions due to a lack of screening modalities i.e., CXR in smokers has resulted in an increased diagnosis of lung cancer by 27% in some reports, even when it was controlled for the previously reported controls. If we stretch our imagination across various disease entities i.e., heart attacks, breast cancer, colon cancer the numbers of undiagnosed and unrecognized will be astronomical.

Infection by Double Mutant Strain

Because of the lack of herd immunity, the virus is rapidly mutating into resistant strains. The B.1.167 strain has been very elusive and is responsible for the second wave and surge of the pandemic. Currently it is responsible for the apocalyptic outbreak in India. Close to half a million people are being infected and two patients were dying every minute during the surge at its peak. It is supposedly evasive to the benefits offered by the currently available vaccines. Similar mutant strains are responsible for outbreaks in the UK (Kent Strains), Brazil and South Africa.

Covid Associated Mucormycosis (CAM)
aka - *Black Fungus*

An emerging phenomenon has been brought to light during the second surge of COVID-19 in India. There is an increased incidence of mucormycosis in patients who were treated for COVID-19 infection. This disease is caused by a group of molds or fungi called mucormycetes. Multiple factors are at hand for identification of this fungal infection since steroids have found a unique niche in the treatment of these patients. But also, there is a higher attack rate of COVID infection in patients with diabetes. Since, steroids are administered at much higher doses by intravenous, oral and inhaled and for prolonged periods of time. If overcrowding, and a hot and humid environment and ubiquitous nature of this fungus is taken into account, then all dots can be connected to factors which have led to an unprecedented surge in mucormycosis. It is a rare yet deadly disease, especially in the vulnerable and susceptible diabetic and immunocompromised patients. Mucormycosis can be rather elusive initially as the presentation is rather subtle and can often go unrecognized. This can be a major problem when resources are stretched too thin and the nation's healthcare delivery is compromised. The symptoms of mucormycosis can range from headache to sinus pressure as ear, nose and throat are first ones to get affected due to humid and moist surfaces. Other signs are eye pain, blurry vision and swollen sinus areas like cheeks and nostrils.

On exam the affected areas appear to be blackened, hence the term "black mold". This deadly disease can have a rather rapid spread to the other organs and systems if not readily diagnosed or treated. It can spread to the brain, especially through sinuses and eyes, if it remains untreated for days. Once, brain is affected the mortality can go more than 50%. Even if the disease doesn't kill you, it will have long term sequelae and consequences with potential disabilities. The treatment of mucormycosis is successful, with early recognition, detection and surgical intervention in combination with the antifungals. There are various antifungals available, but the most prevalent and readily available is prolonged Amphotericin-B. Hygenicity along with multiple other factors also play a role in disease acquisition and progression. Due to unsanitary conditions, along with other predisposing factors i.e., steroids, immunocompromised status, this particular fungus species has been flourishing in Southeast Asia at a rampant pace.

Covid Associated Candidiasis (CAC)
aka - White Fungus

Another emerging and often debilitating condition has emerged in patients who are infected with COVID-19 and are being treated with a prolonged course of steroids and antibiotics. Both steroids and antibiotics make a patient susceptible and vulnerable to opportunistic infections which include various fungi. Mucormycosis is one of those and the other one is candida. *Candida Albicans* and *candida Auris* have emerged as one of the common species. *Candida Auris* is often referred to as white fungus as compared with mucormycosis, which is referred to as black fungus. The white fungus is also denoted as *C. Auris, which* can cause a unique discoloration of the mouth and mucous membranes. This can also result in systemic manifestation of the disease, urinary tract infection, sepsis and bloodstream infections. This infection is often drug resistant and poses a specific threat to immunocompromised hosts, such as diabetics, HIV/AIDS and cancer patients. These fungal infections came to light after a devastating second COVID-19 surge in India. Candida Auris is a relatively new variant of the candida family which has emerged in the past ten years. Once this fungus accesses the bloodstream, it can present a unique diagnostic and treatment dilemma to the treating ICU physicians. Thankfully it only affects 20-30 critically ill patients. The infection is especially pronounced in the patients who are ventilated. Lack of necessary preventive measures, due to multiple factors i.e., lack of PPE, overworked healthcare workers, lack of handwashing, changing gloves and gowns between patients, led to frequent outbreaks of this fungal infection.

COVID Nomenclature
"THE NAME GAME"

It was quite challenging to name variants when they started to emerge at a bristling pace, creating an epidemic within a pandemic. Initially referred to as B.1.1.7 (UK variant) from B.1.351 (South African variant) or B.1.617.2 (Indian variant but was confusing and hard to follow, if not continuing the trend of outright orientalism as the origination point for the virus. However, that nomenclature was also short-sighted, especially when the B.1.617.2 crossed the artificial geographical boundaries and travelled to 80 different countries. The WHO convened a nomenclature committee to alleviate the confusion. This committee, composed of world's greeted healthcare leaders, decided to name the new variant according to the Roman Alphabet Currently B.1.617.2 is termed the "delta" variant. It is rapidly spreading across the globe and has been cultivated in 80 countries, as of the writing of this book. It is more contagious than the first prolific variant and even more deadly. Recent mutations of COVID-19 are emerging by the day, with new ones being titled *"Lambda"* and *"Mu"* variants B.1.621. Hopefully we can reach some sort of herd immunity before we can even think of naming a "Zeta" variant.

CURRENT EVIDENCE-BASED COVID TREATMENT GUIDELINES

Remdesivir is the only FDA approved therapy in COVID-19; other agents are under investigation for the treatment of COVID-19. Treatment efficacy has been demonstrated with length of stay impact by Remdesivir in non-critically ill patients.

RECOVERY - randomized control trials demonstrated that dexamethasone offers mortality benefit in those with acute hypoxemic respiratory failure and CODEX trial demonstrated an increase in ventilator-free days when both used in combination.

CLINICAL	SUPPORTIVE	TARGETED
• Asymptomatic	• Acetaminophen for fever	• None
• Suspected COVID-19 • Shortness of Breath • Spo2<92%	• Acetaminophen • Anticoagulation	• None

• Confirmed COVID-19 • Oxygen Requirement >10 L	• Acetaminophen • Dexamethasone 6 mg daily-10 days OR • Dexamethasone 20 mg daily 20 mg for 5 days and then 10 mg daily • Anticoagulation with Lovenox 30 or 40 mg subcutaneous twice daily OR • Heparin 5000 *IU* TID	SARS-COV 2 antibody negative • casirivimab +imdevimab (regeneron) 600mg/600 x 1
• Confirmed COVID-19 • Requiring >10L NC via heated or non-heated high flow nasal cannula • Requiring Non-invasive ventilation or Invasive mechanical ventilation	• Enoxaparin DVT prophylaxis: 40mg or 30mg BID* Therapeutic anticoagulation NOT recommended unless confirmed VTE • Dexamethasone 6 mg QD x10 days2 or dexamethasone 20 mg QD x 5 days, dexamethasone 10mg x5 days3 • Acetaminophen PRN	• Consider tocilizumab • If tocilizumab not available, consider baricitinib • Sars-COV 2 antibody negative: • Casirivimab + imdevim

ADJUVANT ANTIBIOTICS:
- Co-infections with secondary infections in COVID-19 are only 8% per meta-analysis, therefore empiric use of antibiotics on all COVID-19 patients is not routinely recommended. However, antibiotics for the following conditions can be initiated as indicated at physician discretion.
- Community Acquired Pneumonia (CAP) Ceftriaxone + azithromycin or doxycycline
- Beta-lactam allergy: Levofloxacin
- Gram negative coverage Ceftriaxone OR Cefepime (Pseudomonal coverage) OR meropenem for Extended Spectrum Beta Lactamases (ESBL coverage)
- MRSA – (Methicillin Resistant Staph Aureus) coverage - MRSA nasal PCR for COVID-19 confirmed cases

O Linezolid- preferred if bacteremia is not suspected
O Vancomycin- only if contraindication to linezolid or bacteremia is suspected

CORTICOSTEROIDS:
- RECOVERY trial with dexamethasone 6mg daily x 10 days vs none showed a mortality reduction in patients on supplemental oxygen only
- The CoDEX trial with dexamethasone 20mg daily x 5 days, followed by dexamethasone

10mg daily x 5 days vs none showed a significant increase in ventilator free days over 28 days.
- The CAPE COVID trial evaluated hydrocortisone 200mg daily x 7 days, followed by hydrocortisone 100mg daily x 4 days, then 50mg daily x 3 days (14 total days) vs placebo showed no significant difference in the primary outcome of treatment at 21 days. This study was stopped early and likely underpowered to detect a difference.
- The REMAP-CAP trial, a multicenter open-label trial, randomized patients to hydrocortisone 50mg q6h x 7 days or hydrocortisone 50mg q6h while in shock for up to 28 days, or no intervention. The study was stopped early and therefore, a definitive conclusion cannot be made.

REMDISIVIR:
- The ACTT-1 trial (Remdesivir 200mg x1 day, followed by 100mg x 9 days vs placebo) showed shorter recovery time to recovery in the Remdesivir group, with those on supplemental oxygen benefiting most from therapy.
- The SOLIDARITY trial by the World Health Organization (WHO) did not show any difference in mortality, ventilation initiation, or time to discharge when comparing Remdesivir to its placebo.

- The SIMPLE-1 A randomized, open-label trial, evaluating 5-day vs 10-day courses of Remdesivir showed no significant difference in efficacy when comparing 5- vs 10-day courses after adjustment of disease severity. Of note, only 44% of patients in the 10-day group completed a full course of therapy. Few mechanically ventilated or ECMO patients were included in the analysis.
- The SIMPLE-2, A randomized open-label trial comparing standard of care, up to a 5-day course of Remdesivir, and up to a 10-day course of Remdesivir in patients with moderate COVID-19 in a 1:1:1 fashion. The study found a statistically significant, but not clinically significant, difference in clinical status at day 11 in those receiving a 5-day course of Remdesivir versus standard of care. There was no significant difference in clinical status at day 11 in those receiving a 10-day course of therapy versus standard of care.
- Duration of therapy is 5 total days. There is uncertainty regarding whether Remdesivir confers clinical benefit in patients who require high-flow oxygen, non-invasive ventilation, mechanical ventilation, or ECMO.

BARICITINIB:

- Baricitinib, a selective Janus kinase (JAK) 1 and 2 inhibitor, has been studied for use in combination with or without Remdesivir for COVID-19 infection.
- The CTT-2 trial showed baricitinib 4 mg daily x 14 days or until hospital discharge (or 2 mg daily if CrCl <60mL/min) in combination with Remdesivir was compared to Remdesivir alone. Overall, patients receiving combination therapy recovered about one day sooner than those only receiving Remdesivir. The recovery time benefit of combination therapy was seen most in patients receiving noninvasive ventilation or high-flow oxygen (10 days in combination vs 18 days in the Remdesivir group). Of note, steroids were not a standard of care in the trial, potentially limiting applicability.
- Though baricitinib carries a warning for risk of thrombosis, rates of this adverse event were similar between both groups. Given this risk, consideration of dopplers to evaluate active VTE may be elevated in patients on this therapy in the correct clinical scenario.

TOCILIZUMAB:

- Tocilizumab is an IL-6 inhibitor which has been evaluated for potential impact in patients with severe COVID-19 infection.

- The EMPACTA, phase III trial of tocilizumab in hospitalized patients with severe COVID-19 associated pneumonia showed no improvement in clinical status or mortality.
- The RCT-TCZ-COVID-19 comparing the use of tocilizumab versus usual care in hospitalized patients with COVID-19 pneumonia showed no benefit on disease progression in these patients. In non-ICU patients with moderate to severe COVID-19 pneumonia on oxygen support (CORIMUNO-19)17 tocilizumab was no different than usual care when comparing mortality outcomes.
- The BACC-BAY trial compared tocilizumab versus standard of care in moderately ill hospitalized patients and found no difference in risk of intubation or death. Tocilizumab patients had significantly higher neutropenia and infection.
- A retrospective analysis showed a higher incidence of secondary bacterial infections in patients with COVID-19 receiving tocilizumab versus those who did not receive tocilizumab.1
- The REMAP-CAP is an open label trial that compared tocilizumab or sarilumab versus standard of care in critically ill patients requiring respiratory or cardiovascular organ support. Preliminary results showed higher median organ support-free days with tocilizumab

and sarilumab compared to control (10 vs 11 vs 0 days) as well as a trend toward decrease in mortality (28.0 vs 22.2 vs 35.8%).

- The RECOVERY trial is a randomized, open-label, controlled trial assessing the use of tocilizumab plus usual standard of care (i.e., dexamethasone) versus usual standard of care alone. Patients in the study were included if there was clinical evidence of progressive COVID-19 and had a CRP ³ 7.5 mg/dL. There was a significant reduction in mortality in the tocilizumab group compared to usual care (29% vs 33%). Results are currently pending peer review.

BAMLANIVIMAB+ ETESEVIMAB

- These are recombinant neutralizing human IgG1k monoclonal antibodies which block spike protein attachment of SARS-CoV-2 to human ACE2 receptors.
- The BLAZE-1 trial evaluated Bamlanivimab monotherapy versus bamlanivimab + etesevimab administered as a one-time dose in high-risk patients versus placebo with SARS-CoV-2 in the outpatient setting. Patients were randomized to receive one of three bamlanivimab doses (700mg, 2800mg, 7000mg), combination bamlanivimab + etesevimab (2800mg + 2800mg) or placebo. The trial showed a

- significant reduction in viral load in the combination group when compared to placebo, with potential to decrease hospitalization.
- EUA for bamlanivimab + etesevimab 700mg /1400mg x1 in high-risk outpatients with SARS-CoV-2 (limitations of authorized use outlined by FDA).
- Bamlanivimab is NOT recommended in hospitalized patients as demonstrated by the TICO trial, showing that there was no difference in clinical outcomes at day 5 in hospitalized patients when compared to placebo.

REGENERON - REGN-COV
Antibody Cocktail
- REGN-COV is a combination of monoclonal antibodies (casirivimab and imdevimab) proposed to reduce viral load and symptoms associated with COVID-19 by blocking infectivity of SARS-CoV-2. Currently, a randomized, double-blind trial comparing the addition of REGN-COV versus placebo to standard-of-care is ongoing in both outpatient and inpatient settings.
- Interim analysis from 275 non-hospitalized COVID (+) shows a possible decrease in time to symptom resolution in a subset of patients who did not have measurable antiviral antibodies prior to treatment initiation

- For hospitalized adult patients (≥18 years old) with symptomatic COVID-19, casirivimab 600 mg + imdevimab 600 mg may be considered for inpatient utilization based off results from the RECOVERY trial. Trial results demonstrated that addition of the combination of 2 monoclonal antibodies to usual care resulted in a statistically significant improvement in mortality in seronegative patients at baseline. Allocation to the therapy arm was also associated with a lower risk of progression to mechanical ventilation.

BUDESONIDE:

- The STOIC trial compared inhaled budesonide vs standard of care (SOC) in adult patients with mild COVID-19. A total of 146 patients were included (73 in each arm). Budesonide patients received 800μg (400 μg inhalation x2) twice daily and continued until symptoms resolved.
- The primary outcome evaluated was the rate of COVID-19 related urgent care visits. Primary outcome occurred in 15% of SOC vs 3% for budesonide (p=0.009). Self-reported clinical recovery was 8 days for SOC vs 7 for budesonide (p=0.007).

BROVANA- or FORMOTEROL- LONG-ACTING BETA AGONIST:
- Not formally studied in COVID-19, patients, however, anecdotally proven its robust and significant bronchodilator properties in any bronchospastic or bronchoconstrictor condition. This bronchodilator property renders it a great adjuvant nebulized therapy in conjunction budesonide

MUCOMYST:
- *N. Acetylcysteine* is another mucolytic agent which can be used as a nebulized therapy. It helps "thin up, "or "breakdown" the tenacious mucus which often accompanies COVID-19 pneumonia. Works best when combined with budesonide and brovana.

IVERMECTIN: AKA *"THE HORSE PILL"*
- Ivermectin is an anti-parasitic agent which is used in medicine to treat intestinal worm infestation in both humans (treat tropical diseases such as river blindness, strongyloides etc.) and veterinary medicine animals-pets for deworming. Initially showed some antiviral activity (including SARS-CoV-2) in vitro.
- In a pilot study of 24 patients with non-severe COVID-19, patients were randomized to ivermectin 400mcg/kg x1 vs placebo. There

was no difference in positive PCRs at day 7 post-treatment. There was a reduction in self-reported anosmia, hyposmia, and cough.
- In a single-center, randomized trial evaluating ivermectin x 5 days versus placebo, there was no significant difference in time to resolution of symptoms.
- A meta-analysis of ten randomized controlled trials determined that ivermectin did not decrease mortality, length of stay, decreased need for mechanical ventilation, or respiratory viral clearance.
- The TOGETHER trial, an ongoing randomized adaptive trial to investigate the efficacy of re-purposed treatments for COVID-19 among high-risk adults, demonstrated no benefit to ivermectin (400 mcg/kg) when compared to placebo.

CONVALESCENT PLASMA:
- A double-blind randomized control trial conducted in New York showed no difference in improved outcome when comparing convalescent plasma to standard plasma.

NSAIDs-NON-STEROIDAL ANTI-INFLAMMATORY DRUGS:
- Early reports recommended against the use of NSAIDs due to the possibility of adverse

outcomes. However, no data to validate the observational data has been published.
- Available guidelines have recommended caution with use and clinical judgment but no contraindication to the use of NSAIDS when indicated.

Patients with prior COVID-19 vaccination:
- At this time, no data exists to guide treatment of patients with COVID-19 who previously received a COVID-19 vaccine.
- Currently, a booster shot is recommended in previously vaccinated, immunocompromised individuals.

Pregnancy:
- CDC recommends vaccination during pregnancy

FAST FACTS

COVID-19

Outbreak: 2019 - Ongoing in 2021

Greatest Respiratory pandemic of the modern time

Mortality rate: 150 million people infected, 3.3 million deaths 91 million-recovered

Mode of transmission: human to human, respiratory-aerosolized-droplet-airborne

Symptoms: fever, body ache, chills and loss of taste and smell

Complications: respiratory failure, stroke, heart disease, kidney failure, Pulmonary Embolism

Vaccine: Multiple vaccine available (Pfizer and Moderna have been declared safe for use in Pregnancy)

Diagnosis: Rapid antigen test-PCR-antibody

Treatment: Oxygen-Remdesivir-steroids-convalescent plasma-monoclonal Antibodies, anticoagulation

SPANISH FLU-1918
aka "Gripe Espanola" or "Avian Flu" - H1N1-Flu

DEFINITION:
The first known modern-day pandemic with the highest mortality. This was caused by Influenza A and had a high propensity for being complicated by post viral pneumonia, also known as the flu pandemic of 1918. This started as an Influenza A epidemic after the first world war and lasted for about two years. It infected about 500 million people around the globe and annihilated 5-10 % of the world's population which was around 3 billion people at that time. According to some accounts, 50-100 million people died during that pandemic.

Number of cases: 500 million cases, roughly 1/3 of the world's population at that time which was 3 billion in 1918.

Number of Deaths: 50-100 million in the world, 675,000 in the USA.

Period: Jan 1918-Dec 1920.

EPIDEMIOLOGY
A negative single stranded RNA virus which belongs to the family of *Orthomyxoviridae*. These viruses are prevalent during the winter and annually are responsible for about 30,000 cases across the US. However,

this antigenically novel virus was the first of its kind which caused the pandemic of 1918.

Background
The term Spanish Flu has nothing to do with Spain, as this was the only country which was not involved in the First World War. Therefore, its media and government did not have any reservations in publishing the true number of cases, mortality and the pandemic nature of it, while the other nations were trying to downplay the impact of it. Flu of 1918 was spread by the birds and hence called "Avian Flu" or "Bird Flu." In biological terms, it was called H1N1 Flu. The first letter "H" denotes the enzymatic particle, hemagglutinin and the second letter "N" as neuraminidase. The numbers "1-23 etc." connotes changes in the arrangement and rearrangement of these glycoproteins. This rearrangement is what caused various outbreaks time and again.

Host: direct contact from chicken to human.

Transmission
The virus can spread from a human to human via direct contact and or as a droplet transmission. This means that the virus can spread via physical contact with another human as well as through the inhalation of respiratory droplets which become aerosolized or airborne during the cough, sneeze of an infected person. Swine has been implicated and proposed as a

"mixing vessel" intermediary host between birds and humans in later pandemics of 1957 and 1968 (Am J of Epidemiology, -Dec 2018). There is proposed bi-directional transmissibility between swine-humans.

INCUBATION PERIOD:
24-48 hours.

SIGNS AND SYMPTOMS (1ST WAVE, SPRING 1918)
Common viral symptoms occurred including fever, chills, cough, and fatigue. People tend to recover quickly with a very low death rate.

SIGNS AND SYMPTOMS (2ND WAVE, FALL 1918)
People presented with severe URI symptoms including fever, chills, cough, cyanosis of fingers/toes/lips. Hypoxia was rapid in onset and people were progressing to signs of shock (tachycardia, hypotension, tachypnea, mottling) within hours of presentation.

Also, there was a big push for the use of aspirin for symptomatic treatment due to its ability to lower fever and alleviate body aches. The guidelines, at that time, recommended upwards of 30 grams of aspirin a day (keep in mind, we recommend no more than 4grams per day now). Unfortunately, due to this practice many people were presenting with aspirin poisoning- hyperventilation, altered mental status, severe pulmonary edema- and it is estimated that many of the deaths during the second wave were due to aspirin poisoning.

Similar analogy will be hydroxychloroquine, which was pushed initially during COVID-19 infection, which resulted in increased morbidity and mortality.

TREATMENT:
Symptomatic
Aspirin for fever and body aches. Fluids for dehydration. Antibiotics for pneumonia, which was suspected to be bacterial in nature at that time.

Blood transfusions
physicians at the time found that outcomes were improved when blood products were taken from Spanish flu survivors and transfused into high risk for mortality patients who had contracted the Spanish flu complicated by pneumonia. Mortality was 59% if the blood was transfused after 4 days whereas mortality was 19% if the blood was transfused within 4 days.

INTERESTING FACTS:
Also known as the 3-day fever, it is responsible for 50-100 million deaths across the world.

Symptoms also included coughing blood and bleeding from the nose and eyes.

Mode of transmission: chicken to humans, but pigs can catch both human and avian flu.

CORONAVIRUS AKA COVID-19 - SARS-COV-2

FAST FACTS

Outbreak: 1918-1920
Greatest Flu
Mortality rate: 50-100 million people worldwide
Mode of transmission: human to human
Symptoms: fever, body ache, chills and loss of appetite
Complications: respiratory failure and death

ASIAN FLU (1956-1958)
aka H2N2 Flu

DEFINITION:
A pandemic of influenza A (H2N2) in 1957-58. First identified in China in late February 1957, the Asian flu spread to the United States by June 1957 where it caused about 70,000 deaths. It is also known as *Asian influenza*.

Number of cases: Case-fatality rate was reported to be 0.2% by WHO. As per this, the total number of cases can be estimated around 2 billion (which was about ⅔ of the world population at the time).

Number of Deaths: 2 million worldwide and 70,000 in the USA.

Period: 1956-1958.

Epidemiology: Caused by Influenza A-H2N2 subtype. In the 1960s, the human H2N2 strain underwent a series of minor genetic modifications, a process known as antigenic drift. These slight modifications produced periodic epidemics. After 10 years of evolution, the 1957 flu virus disappeared, having been replaced through an antigenic shift by a new influenza A subtype, H3N2, which gave rise to the 1968 flu pandemic.

CORONAVIRUS AKA COVID-19 - SARS-COV-2

Geography: Originated in Guizhou province of China and travelled across to the USA, via Singapore and Hong Kong.

Host: Humans.

Transmission: Person to person by direct contact or droplets.

Incubation period: 1-4 days.

Signs and Symptoms: Presentation ranging from mild upper respiratory infection (fever and cough) to rapid progression to severe pneumonia, acute respiratory distress syndrome, shock and even death.

VACCINATION:
- Live attenuated vaccine (Intranasal spray).
- Inactivated vaccine (Intramuscular).

TREATMENT:
Symptomatic
- Acetaminophen for fever and body aches.
- Fluids for dehydration
- Antibiotics for pneumonia, which was suspected to be bacterial in nature at that time.

The rapid development of a vaccine limited the spread and mortality of the pandemic.

THE NEW PANDEMIC

FAST FACTS

Outbreak: 1956-1958
Dr. Maurice Hilleman, Chief of respiratory disease at Walter Reed army institute of research studied Antigenic drift and helped develop the Vaccine for Asian flu among 40 other vaccines that he developed
Mortality rate: 2 million people worldwide
Mode of transmission: mutation in wild ducks and preexisting human strain
Symptoms: fever, body ache, chills and loss of appetite
Complications included dehydration, seizures, heart failure and death

FLU PANDEMIC (1968)
aka "Hong Kong Flu" - H2N3 Flu

DEFINITION:
The 1968 pandemic was caused by an influenza A (H3N2) virus comprised of two genes from an avian influenza A virus, including a new H3 hemagglutinin, but also contained the N2 neuraminidase from the 1957 H2N2 virus. It was first noted in the United States in September 1968.

Number of cases: It was the third flu epidemic of the century which lasted 2 years from 1968-1970 and afflicted upwards of tens and millions of people.

Number of Deaths: One million to four million worldwide, 500,000 in Hong Kong (15% of its population at that time) and 100,000 in the USA.

Period: July 1968-1970.

Epidemiology: Influenza A, H3N2 subtype (low infectivity rate).

Geography: First reported in Hong Kong in July 1968 and spread like a wildfire within a couple of weeks and spread to Singapore, Vietnam, Philippines, Europe and the USA.

Host: Humans.

Transmission: Person to person by direct contact or droplets.

Incubation period: 1-4 days.

SIGNS AND SYMPTOMS:
- Mild upper respiratory infection fever and cough
- Severe pneumonia
- Acute respiratory distress syndrome
- Shock and even death.

VACCINATION:
- Even though a vaccine was developed, it was too late in the epidemic.
- Live attenuated vaccine (Intranasal spray).
- Inactivated vaccine (Intramuscular).

TREATMENT:
Symptomatic.
- Acetaminophen for fever and body aches.
- Fluids for dehydration.
- Antibiotics for pneumonia, which was initially suspected to be bacterial in nature at that time.

CORONAVIRUS AKA COVID-19 - SARS-COV-2

FAST FACTS

Outbreak: 1968
3rd Major Flu pandemic of the century
Mortality rate: 2-4 million people worldwide
Mode of transmission: human to human-droplet
Symptoms: fever, body ache, chills and loss of appetite
Complications: respiratory failure and death

AVIAN FLU
aka Bird Flu-H1N1-pdm09

DEFINITION:
A contagious respiratory illness, which spreads through aerosolized droplet infection, from animals and humans. There was less common spread through contact with the infected surfaces. The flu epidemic of 2009 closely resembles that of 1918 and has the same nomenclature H1N1.

Number of cases: 60 million cases.

Number of Deaths: 12,469 in the USA, approximately 150,000-500,000 globally.

Period: April 2009-April 2010.

EPIDEMIOLOGY:
This virus was quite different from the already circulating strain in 2019, hence was named the novel virus H1N1-pdm09. It affected the younger population, who did not have immunity against this virus. Populations who were older than 60 years were spared due to pre-existing immunity. Another sub-group of patients who were more susceptible was the pregnant.

Host: non-human reservoir-North American Swine.

CORONAVIRUS AKA COVID-19 - SARS-COV-2

Transmission: Swine to Humans and Humans to Humans.

Incubation period: 1-4 days, however the infected person can remain contagious for a week.

SIGNS AND SYMPTOMS:
It presents as a respiratory infection.

Mild Symptoms:
- Fever
- Cough
- Shortness of breath
- Nausea, vomiting, Diarrhea

Severe Disease: Manifests in patients with underlying comorbid conditions:
- Respiratory Failure
- Pneumonia
- Acute Respiratory Distress Syndrome (ARDS)

Vaccination: H1N1 vaccine.

TREATMENT:
- Symptomatic and supportive treatment.
- Oseltamivir.
- Zanamivir.
- Ventilator support.

- ECMO-in severe or refractory cases improved clinical outcomes.
- Antibiotics for patients who had co-existent or superimposed bacterial infection.

FAST FACTS

Outbreak: 2009-10
Bird Flu-H1N1-mimics the flu pandemic of 1918
Mortality rate: 150,000 million people worldwide
Mode of transmission: human to human
Population Affected: Young Population-Pregnant
Symptoms: fever, body ache, chills
Complications: respiratory failure and death
Treatment: ECMO was quite successful

SARS-CoV
Severe Acute Respiratory Syndrome

Definition:
Quite literally a cousin of the COVID-19, severe acute respiratory syndrome (SARS) is a viral respiratory illness caused by a coronavirus called SARS-associated coronavirus (SARS-CoV) vs. SARS-CoV-2, which is the virus which causes COVID-19. SARS-CoV was first reported in Asia in February 2003. The illness spread to more than two dozen countries in North America, South America, Europe, and Asia before the SARS global outbreak of 2003 was contained.

Number of cases: 8422 cases.

Number of Deaths: 916 deaths.

Period: 2002-2004.

Geography
In 2002-2003, an epidemic occurred in China which primarily affected the respiratory system.

Epidemiology
Coronavirus originated in China and quickly spread across the globe. It purportedly came from an unknown animal source. Civet cats or bats have been implicated as the host reservoir. The index case was

thought to have come from Guangdong province of southern China in 2002. This epidemic spread across 26 countries and affected about 8,000 people worldwide. After the initial acquisition of the virus from the animal host, the rapid spread occurred due to human-to-human transmission of the disease. Most cases of disease transmission are due to lab accidents rather than any other mode of transmission. However other modes of transmission i.e., consumption of the infected animals' meat has been implicated in contracting and transmission of the disease.

INCUBATION PERIOD
2-7 days but can last up to 10 days.

CLINICAL SYMPTOMS-COURSE
It initially presented as either a subtle upper respiratory symptom or flagrant and full-blown pneumonia. There were also constitutional symptoms, which are associated with SARS including fever, chills and myalgia. The symptom complex consists of cough, shortness of breath to pneumonia and respiratory failure. Hypoxia was one of the most common clinical findings. Pneumonia often resulted in severe acute respiratory syndrome, or SARS for short.

DIAGNOSIS
Often clinical depending on the symptoms in the epidemic area. Lab findings of coronavirus were

MERS
Middle Eastern Respiratory Syndrome aka "Camel Fever"

DEFINITION
It is an acute respiratory infection which causes a myriad of respiratory illnesses ranging from upper respiratory tract infection to pneumonia. It was initially described as Middle Eastern Respiratory Syndrome (MERS) and kept the same nomenclature when it spread as an epidemic. It originated *de novo* in the Kingdom of Saudi Arabia.

Number of cases: 2468 cases.

Number of Deaths: 858 deaths.

Period: 2012-Present. Case spike in 2014. The number of cases has dwindled.

EPIDEMIOLOGY
It was considered a novel *beta-coronavirus*, which presented as an outbreak in 2012. It spread to quite a few countries beyond its point of origin in Saudi Arabia. MERS became quiescent within a short span of time. The risk of spread to the global population remains relatively low at this juncture.

confirmatory, though not needed to establish the diagnosis.

TREATMENT
Mostly supportive, ranging from simple hydration to oxygenation. Intensive care was often needed for severely ill patients who required full mechanical ventilatory support.

DURATION OF ILLNESS
3-6 weeks in most cases.

PROPHYLAXIS - PREVENTION
None recommended as there is a very low risk of infectivity or transmission.

FAST FACTS

Outbreak: 2003
CORONA - COVID-19's Cousin
Origin: China
Mortality rate: Few thousand people worldwide
Mode of transmission: human to human - respiratory
Symptoms: fever, body ache, chills and loss of appetite
Complications: respiratory failure and death

CORONAVIRUS AKA COVID-19 - SARS-COV-2

ETIOLOGY
It was caused by beta-coronavirus, which is a single stranded RNA virus.

VECTORS/HOSTS
Bats, camels and humans were thought to be the common vectors for this virus. Infections occurred when in close contact with bats or camels.

CLINICAL MANIFESTATION
It presents primarily as a respiratory infection, which can range from mild to severe disease.

Mild Symptoms:
- Fever
- Cough
- Shortness of breath
- Nausea, vomiting, Diarrhea

Severe Disease
- Manifests in patients with underlying comorbid conditions
- Respiratory Failure
- Pneumonia

MORTALITY
One third of the confirmed diagnosed patients will die, which is quite significant i.e., very high "Case Fatality Rate."

Treatment

There is no currently available vaccine. The treatment is often symptomatic with supportive care. However, vigorous hand washing, droplet precautions and minimizing contact with the infected animal, i.e., camel in this case, is highly recommended.

FAST FACTS
Outbreak: 2012-14 CORONA Origin: Arabian Peninsula Mortality rate: Few thousand people worldwide High Mortality Rate Mode of transmission: human to human - respiratory Symptoms: fever, body ache, chills and Pneumonia Complications: respiratory failure and death

LASSA FEVER
aka *"Lassamammarena Virus"* - *LASV*

DEFINITION
A zoonotic viral disease that results in hemorrhagic manifestation, i.e., gut bleeding when a healthy person or a host comes in contact with an infected person or rodents. Multimammate rat *Mastocytes natalensis* is a common host and carrier of this disease. These infected rats often spread the disease through bodily secretions i.e., urine or excrements i.e., droppings. Lassa fever's clinical presentation mimics that of the Ebola *Virus or Marburg Virus.*

Etiology: Caused by *Lassa Mammaarena Virus,* which belongs to the family of *arena viruses* which causes Viral Hemorrhagic Fever (VHF), first identified in *Lassa* Nigeria in 1969

Number of cases: 100,000 - 300,000 cases annually.

Number of Deaths: 5000 deaths annually.

Period: 1950-Present.

INCUBATION PERIOD
1-3 weeks after coming in contact with an infected rodent or human.

High Risk Patients
- Pregnant-3rd trimester.
- Healthcare workers.
- Unsanitary and overcrowded living conditions.

Transmission: Person to person is less common, but when it does, it is due to contact with blood, mucus or through sexual transmission. Healthcare workers are more susceptible, as the first few cases were reported in the missionary nurses providing care for the pregnant patients in Lassa, Nigeria. Humans get infected when coming into contact with infected rat droppings or urine through contact with food, water and air conditioning units. The virus can be transmitted via semen up to 3 months.

Clinical Symptoms
Asymptomatic   80%
Symptomatic   20%
- Fever
- Bleeding or hemorrhage in mucous membranes or from the gut
- Deafness is often permanent
- Pregnant in third semester are more susceptible

Epidemiology
This viral disease is endemic to West African countries i.e., Nigeria, Sierra Leone, Guinea and Liberia. The case fatality rate is 23%.

Diagnosis
- Antigen Testing
- Antibody Testing (ELISA)
  - Ig-G
  - Ig-M
- Culture
- PCR
- Immunohistochemistry stains

Treatment
Ribavirin if given early.

Supportive:
- Oxygen and ventilatory support.
- Fluid and electrolyte replacements.
- Blood Products.

Complications
- Acute Hearing loss (Deafness 20-30%).
- Stillbirth (when contracted during the third trimester) - 95%.

Prognosis
- 15% out-patient.
- 65% in-patient.

Vaccine
Not available.
Ribavirin can be used prophylactically and empirically.

Prevention

- Universal precautions - travelers and health-care workers.
- Hand hygiene - washing hands with soap and water.
- Barrier precautions when working in close proximity to patients.
- Proper PPE (gloves, masks).
- Proper disposal of the waste.
- Safe lab handling of the specimens.
- Safe mortuary practices.

FAST FACTS

Outbreak: 1950
Ebola's Cousin
Origin: Africa
Mortality rate: Few thousand people worldwide annually
Mode of transmission: Rats - human to human
- respiratory
Symptoms: fever, body ache, chills and loss of appetite
Complications: bleeding and death
Wash all cans containing food and beverage before consumption

EBOLA VIRUS
aka "Ebola Hemorrhagic Fever" EHF or "Ebola Virus Disease" EVD

DEFINITION
Ebola Virus Disease or EVD, is a disease endemic to the sub-Saharan desert region of Africa. This disease manifests as profuse and profound hemorrhage when a healthy person comes in contact with an infected human or a rodent. Ebola is a virus, which was first recognized on the world's stage as an outbreak in 2014-16.

Number of cases: 28,600 cases reported from 2014-2016 (Most severe outbreak of Ebola) with 11 cases reported in the United States.

Number of Deaths: 11,325 deaths reported from 2014-2016 (Most severe outbreak of Ebola).

Period: 1976 - Present. Total 11 outbreaks to date from time to time in several African countries. With the 2014-2016 outbreak being the most severe.

ETIOLOGY
Ebola is a single stranded virus, simply termed EBOV. This genus of *filoviridae* has five strains i.e., Ziare, Sudan, Bundibugyo, Tai Forest, Reston.

Epidemiology

Ebola virus was first discovered as a deadly disease in 1976, near the Ebola River or *"Black River"*, near *Yambuku*, hence the name Ebola virus. The epidemic was first recognized in the Western Africa, in Sierra Leone, Guinea and Liberia. Mortality associated with this epidemic during these two years was slightly less than 12,000 per CDC released data. There have been multiple smaller outbreaks in the western African hemisphere since 1976 but remained fairly small and endemic in the regions. These were contained with the help of local and international healthcare communities. There was an Ebola scare in the United States, after an infected healthcare worker travelled from the endemic area. However, the worker was contained by the establishment of stricter guidelines, which improved quarantine practices in the Ebola task force. These protocols also prepared hospitals and FEMA on training and acquiring proper PPE.

Vectors

The disease is transmitted when a healthy person or animal comes in contact with the secretions of infected humans, rodents, bats, pigs or non-primates i.e., monkeys, gorillas and chimpanzees.

Spread of Disease

It can occur from animals to humans or vice versa. This transmission occurs with contact with the blood, secretions or tissues of an infected human or animal. There are some dietary practices in that part of the world when these infected animals gain access to the food chain. Also, human to human transmission occurs when a diseased infected person is kissed goodbye before burial and there is accidental transfer of the virus to the healthy person. There could also be accidental lab contact. The virus gains access through the broken skin surface or mucous membranes. The virus can remain viable in the body fluids i.e., human semen of an infected person.

PATHOGENESIS

After gaining entry and access through broken surfaces and mucous membranes, the virus hides in the lymph nodes, spleen and liver. The lymphocytosis that occurs with Ebola infection is a result of apoptotic death of the lymphocytes which harbor and carry these viruses and their progeny. The coagulation cascade and supplies are severely impacted due to deleterious effects of the virus on hepatocytes. This is why patients infected with Ebola virus have hemorrhagic manifestation. There is also relative adrenal insufficiency resulting in damage to the zona fasciculata resulting in hypotension and shock. There is a cytokine storm that results in massive release of cytokines, causing capillary leak syndrome and ultimate multi-organ failure.

Clinical Symptoms and Course
- Fever - sudden onset
- Malaise
- Myalgia
- Skin bruising
- Desquamative rash
- Diarrhea and vomiting
- Hemorrhage (most feared and mortal sign and complication of the disease)
- Neurological manifestation including seizure
- Hiccups
- Miscarriage in pregnant women

Incubation
9-11 days.

Diagnosis
Ebola viral load can be detected three days after a person becomes infected.

Blood samples can be tested for the virus via PCR- Polymerase Chain Reaction.

Lab Findings
- Lymphopenia
- Neutrophilic leukocytosis with a left shift
- Thrombocytopenia
- Elevated amylase
- AST>ALT

CORONAVIRUS AKA COVID-19 - SARS-COV-2

- Disseminated Intravascular Coagulation - DIC
- Prolonged PT/PTT
- Elevated Fibrinogen Degradation/Split Product - FDP or FSP
- Elevated D-Dimer

TREATMENT
- Isolation
- Symptomatic
  - Fluid resuscitation
  - Vasopressors for hypotension and shock
  - Correction of electrolytes
  - Blood transfusions as needed
  - Correction of coagulation profile
  - Supplemental oxygen
  - Ventilatory support as needed
  - Nutritional support
  - Managing underlying comorbid conditions
  - Broad spectrum antibiotics if super-infection with bacteria is suspected

There is no antiviral therapy currently available to treat Ebola virus disease EVD. There are a few experimental vaccines available under strict experimental guidelines for the confirmed case.

Cause of death
- Hemorrhagic shock
- Septic shock
- Multi-organ failure

Vaccine

There is a single dose vaccine available called rVSV-ZEBOV- that doesn't cause Ebola infection because it does not contain the whole Ebola virus. Continue with PPE, as the vaccine is not 100% effective.

The infected person can develop an immune response resulting in antibodies, which can render protection for a period of 10 years.

FAST FACTS

Outbreak: 1950
Lassa Fever's Cousin
Origin: Africa
Mortality rate: Few thousand people worldwide annually
Mode of transmission: Rats - human to human - bodily secretions
Symptoms: fever, bleeding
Complications: bleeding and death
Avoid contact with the secretions of the person infected with Ebola
Movie: "Outbreak"

HANTAVIRUS

DEFINITION
A disease spread by rats, causing respiratory tract infection ranging from mild "Flu Like" symptoms to severe pneumonia. Often a forgotten virus, it came back into the limelight a few times, when there was an outbreak in the recent past. To differentiate the disease manifestation in North America from its African counterpart it is called "New World" Hantavirus.

Number of cases: There have been 728 cases of reported hantavirus infections in the US and 2 cases outside the US.

Number of Deaths: The case fatality rate is 36% which estimates about 262 deaths.

Period: 1993-present.

EPIDEMIOLOGY
This is a single stranded RNA virus, which belongs to *Bunyavirus*. There are various strains of hantavirus which take host in species of rodents. Two major outbreaks in 2012, the Seoul Virus and 2017 in Yosemite National Park.

Host

Rodents are the most common host and are responsible for transmission of the disease to humans. This phenomenon occurs when a human comes in direct contact with the virus through secretions from the host such as fresh rat urine, droppings or when rodents become part of the human food chain.

Each *hanta virus* serotype, also known as strain, has a specific rodent host for the specific serotype.

The Cotton Rat *"sigmodon hispidus"* carries the Hanta Virus serotype Black Creek Canal Virus (BCCV).

The Deer Mouse "*Peromyscus maniculatus*" carries the Hanta Virus serotype Sin Nombre.

The Rice Rat *"Oryzomys palustris"* carries the Hanta Virus serotype Bayou Virus (BAYV).

The White-footed Mouse *"Peromyscus leucopus"* carries the Hanta Virus serotype, New York Virus (NYV).

Transmission

This disease is spread from the rodent host to humans via aerosolized virus that is shed from the rodents' excreta such as urine, feces, and saliva. Viruses can also be transmitted via the bite of an infected rodent.

Direct contact: secretions, urine, droppings or tissues or aerosol.

Indirect Transmission:
- Airborne transmission
- Transmission from old uninhibited barns, building in rural settings, especially in rodent infested areas
- Construction workers who work in the crawl spaces, basements and with demolitions
- Hiking and camping can also get exposed to these viruses

Human to Human Transmission
For the most part there is no transmission, however a few case reports have been reported.

Clinical Symptoms
Generalized symptoms - Flu Like Symptoms
- Fever, chills
- Nausea, vomiting, diarrhea
- Headaches, dizziness

Severe Disease
Hantavirus Pulmonary Syndrome (HPS)
- Early HPS includes fever, fatigue, muscle aches, headaches, dizziness, chills, nausea, vomiting, or diarrhea.
- Late HPS starts 4-10 days after the initial phase and includes cough, shortness of breath, chest tightness, sensation of lungs filling with fluid.

Hemorrhagic Fever with Acute Renal Syndrome
- Symptoms develop 1-2 weeks after exposure but can take up to 8 weeks.
- Sudden onset of severe headaches, back and abdominal pain, fever, chills, nausea, blurred vision, flushing of the face, acute shock as seen by hypotension and renal failure with fluid overload.

INCUBATION PERIOD
1-8 weeks.

MORTALITY
38% when HPS sets in and causes severe respiratory failure and death.

DIAGNOSIS
Hantavirus in general is diagnosed by its clinical signs and symptoms, in the right geographical and clinical context.

HFRS can be confirmed with clinical history, evidence of hantavirus antigen in tissue by immunohistochemical staining, or evidence of the hantavirus RNA in blood or tissue.

TREATMENT
There is no specific treatment, vaccine or cure for hantavirus disease.

Supportive therapy is the mainstay and can include

management of hydration status, electrolyte replacement, oxygen therapy and even ventilatory support if evidence of hypoxia is noted, blood pressure support in the setting of shock, and in some instances dialysis when severe fluid overload has occurred.

IV *ribavirin* has been shown to decrease death associated with HFRS if used early in the disease process.

FAST FACTS

Outbreak: 1993
Ebola's Cousin
Origin: Africa and North America
Mortality rate: Few thousand people worldwide annually
Mode of transmission: Rats - human to human - respiratory
Symptoms: fever, bleeding and kidney failure
Complications: bleeding and death
Wash all cans containing food and beverage before consumption

YELLOW FEVER

DEFINITION
Yellow fever is an acute viral illness caused by *flavivirus* in Sub-Saharan Africa and South America. Yellow Fever is transmitted by mosquitoes.

Number of cases: 200,000 cases annually.

Number of Deaths: 30,000 deaths annually.

Period: First epidemic reported in 1648 with multiple outbreaks after that. Currently >90% of the cases are within the African subcontinent.

EPIDEMIOLOGY
It is endemic to Africa and is also prevalent in South America. It is caused by the RNA virus from the genus *flavivirus*.

HOST
- Humans
- Primates

VECTOR
- Mosquito *Aedes of Haemagogus*

INCUBATION PERIOD
5 days.

Clinical Symptoms
The name yellow fever emanates from fever associated with jaundice or yellow skin.

Yellow Fever Stages
   Infection

Initial phase of constitutional symptoms for viremia: Fever and malaise.
   Remission
      Asymptomatic for 48 hours.
   Intoxication

Sequelae of organ dysfunction, hepatic failure, coagulopathy and bleeding.

Treatment
There is no specific cure, but supportive or symptomatic treatment is the only option once symptom complex ensues.

Vaccine
A single dose of vaccine confers lifelong immunity to yellow fever virus. It is a live attenuated vaccine; therefore it should be avoided in pregnancy.

Prevention
- DEET
- Permethrin impregnated clothes

- Proper attire, includeing long sleeve shirts and long pants

---

FAST FACTS

Outbreak: first known in the 1600's anecdotal evidence
Origin: Africa
Mortality rate: 20,000-30,000 people worldwide annually
Mode of transmission: mosquito - primates (intermediate hosts)
Symptoms: fever, yellow skin (jaundice)
Complications: viral hemorrhagic fever-hepatic dysfunction-coagulopathy
Use DEET, permethrin for prevention - vaccine (one dose) lifelong immunity
Avoid yellow fever vaccine during Pregnancy

AIDS
Acquired Immune Deficiency Syndrome

DEFINITION
It is a chronic infectious multiorgan disease complex caused by the HIV-Human Immunodeficiency Virus.

Number of cases: currently about 35 million people are living with HIV/AIDS.

Number of Deaths: 36 million.

Period: First reported in 1976 in Democratic Republic of Congo but peaked around the globe in 2005-2012.

Geography: Even though it is a widespread infection, the majority of HIV positive patients live in Sub-Saharan Africa. Some estimates show 5% infectivity that surmounts to about 21 million people. Due to targeted therapy and intense involvement of the WHO there has been a steady decline in the number of new cases and as a result the mortality due to AIDS has significantly decreased.

CLINICAL MANIFESTATION
It can present with some non-specific signs and symptoms.

Early-onset to 6 months
- Asymptomatic infection may be seen earlier in the course of disease
- Rapid unintentional weight loss
- Recurrent fevers and night sweats
- Lymph node swelling

Late-opportunistic infections-Beyond six months
It can also present later with a variety of illnesses and syndromes including:

Gastrointestinal
Diarrhea is caused by cryptosporidium, pancreatitis, hepatitis.

Neurological
Cryptococcal meningitis, aseptic meningitis, encephalopathy, seizures, Guillain-Barre Syndrome.

Pulmonary
PJP/PCP pneumonia, pneumonitis.

Fungal infections
Oral-genital ulcers and thrush, candidiasis.

Viral illness
Patients with AIDS are susceptible to other viral infections, such as HSV, VZV

Cancer
: Kaposi's sarcoma, lymphoma and some lung cancers have been implicated in AIDS patients. There is an increased predilection of certain other cancers in HIV/AIDS over the years.

DIAGNOSIS

Risk Factors
- All high-risk populations should be screened
- Any new STD-sexually transmitted disease
- LGBTQ men.
- Transexual and high risk heterosexual groups
- Healthcare works with exposure
- Children born to HIV positive mothers
- High risk pregnancy, sex workers or rape cases

Lab testing includes;
- Antigen/antibody immunoassay-HIV antibody/p24 antigen
- Viral load
  Early>100, 000 copies/ml-to millions-highly infectious
  Late 30,000-50,000-low infectivity
- CD-4 count decreases
- CD-8 count increase

Differential Diagnosis
Constellation of initial symptom complexes, especially earlier in the disease process and the presentation resembles infectious mononucleosis-EBV, syphilis, toxoplasmosis. In other words, HIV virus shares its mimicry with other disseminated viral syndromic prodromes.

Treatment
Antiretroviral Therapy (ART) helps maintain disease under control and keeps viral load to sub-clinical level. There is no cure for HIV/AIDS.

Multiple agents, usually three agents, need to be started at the same time to reduce resistance and better tolerability.

Once initiated, ART should continue for a lifetime.

Epidemiology
Prevalent throughout the world, this disease is spread by sexual transmission and coming in contact with bodily secretions. There is also accidental transmission in the healthcare workers by needle. This virus can also be transmitted to newborn children, also through breast milk.

Mortality
Caused by opportunistic infections, which result from the weakened immune system.

CORONAVIRUS AKA COVID-19 - SARS-COV-2

FAST FACTS
Outbreak:1976
Origin: Congo Africa
Mortality rate: 35-35 million (deaths-living with AIDS)
Mode of transmission: Sexual, needles, vertical (maternal-fetal)
Symptoms: non-specific to AIDS-defining illness, PJP (PCP) etc.
Complications: opportunistic infections
Treatment: Highly successful with Antiretroviral therapy - prophylaxis available for high-risk persons

ZIKA VIRUS

Definition
Zika virus got its name from the African forest "Zika," where it was first identified. Zika virus disease is caused by a virus transmitted primarily by *Aedes* mosquitoes, which bites during the day versus its cousin *Anopheles,* which tends to bite in the evening or at night

Number of cases: >92,000 cases.

Number of Deaths: No deaths have yet been reported. However, an 8.3% case fatality rate was reported in infants who develop microcephaly (Zika virus has been associated with microcephaly).

Period: First identified in monkeys in 1947 and in humans in 1952. First major outbreak in 2013.

Epidemiology
It is prevalent in Africa, Asia, Caribbean and South America. It is endemic in more than 100 countries around the world. Infants and pregnancy are particularly at a highest risk of infection and disease manifestation.

Etiology
Zika virus was first identified in *Rhesus monkeys* in the Zika forest in Africa in 1947.

Vector
Aedes Mosquito.

Transmission
- Through the saliva of the infected mosquito bite
- Organ transplantation from the infected person
- Blood or blood products transfusion

Incubation period
2-14 days.

Prevention
Prevention seems to be the best strategy like avoiding mosquito bites, wearing protective clothing or avoiding travel to the endemic areas, especially when pregnant or planning a pregnancy. Zika virus can be passed from a pregnant woman to her fetus. Infection during pregnancy is associated with certain birth defects like microcephaly. It can also be passed through sexual transmission, from a person who has zika to his or her sexual partners. Condoms can reduce the chance of getting Zika through sexual transmission.

Vaccine

No vaccine is currently available. There has been some research underway to make a vaccine for the Zika virus.

Treatment

Symptomatic.

FAST FACTS

Outbreak: first known in the 1940's Major outbreak in 2013
Origin: Africa-South America-Caribbean
Mortality rate: <100,00
Mode of transmission: mosquito
Symptoms: mostly asymptomatic - pregnancy high risk
Complications: microcephaly
Use DEET, permethrin for prevention - No vaccine - Avoid Travel to endemic areas

DENGUE FEVER

DEFINITION
Another cousin of Zika virus and yellow fever, which is spread by an infected mosquito bite and causes bleeding tendency in the infected host, which can result in hemorrhaging.

Number of cases: About 390 million infections occur annually, out of which 96 million manifest clinically and the rest of the cases remain symptom free.

Number of Deaths: About 22,000 deaths are reported annually.

Period: 1950-Present.

EPIDEMIOLOGY
It is prevalent in Africa, Asia. Dengue fever has been reported in more than 100 countries around the world. Infants and pregnancy are particularly at highest risk of infections and associated complications.

ETIOLOGY
This disease is caused by a single-stranded *Dengue* Virus which belongs to the *Flavivirus* genus. There are four serotypes of Dengue Virus i.e., DENV-1 DENV-2, DENV-3 and DENV-4.

Vector
Aedes mosquito.

Transmission
- Through the bite and saliva of the infected mosquito
- Organ transplantation from an infected person
- Blood or blood products transfusion

Incubation Period
Average 4-7 days, up to 15 days.

Clinical Manifestation
- Majority of the patients are asymptomatic or present with mild disease.
- Nausea, vomiting and abdominal pain.
- Bleeding from mucosal membranes.
- Enlarged liver.
- Fever.
- Thrombocytopenia-low platelets.
- *Dengue hemorrhagic fever* (DHF) is the most feared and devastating complication of dengue virus, which presents with bleeding diathesis.
- As with other viral infections, there is a chance to get re-infected especially when the acquired immunity is not as robust or is compromised due to underlying cancer, chemotherapy or other immune deficiency disorders.

- *Dengue Shock Syndrome* (DSS), which can present with profound hypotension and hemodynamic collapse.
- Brain edema, brain hemorrhage and encephalopathy can also occur in susceptible individuals.
- Metabolic Acidosis.

Diagnosis
- Clinical symptoms in the affected geographical location.
- Blood testing for confirmation.

Treatment
- Symptomatic, rest, hydration, acetaminophen.
- Targeted therapy for underlying complications, which may include oxygen, ventilator, transfusion of blood products.

Vaccine
Dengvaxia approved 2019: Three doses are required to induce immunity.

Prevention
- Integrated Mosquito Management.
- Aerial spray.
- Control of standing water-followed by spray.
- DEET.
- Mathurin impregnated clothes.
- Full sleeve shirts and long pants.

FAST FACTS

Outbreak: first known in the 1940's Major outbreak in 2013
Origin: Africa-South America-Caribbean
Mortality rate: <22,000
High Infectivity >400,000 million cases worldwide
Mode of transmission: mosquito
Symptoms: mostly asymptomatic
Complications: hemorrhagic manifestations
Use DEET, permethrin for prevention - vaccine available
- Avoid Travel to endemic areas
Avoid Aspirin and NSAIDS

CHIKUNGUNYA VIRUS

Definition
It is a mosquito borne illness that is spread to humans through the bite of an infected mosquito. Chikungunya virus was first described during an outbreak in Tanzania in 1952. This virus belongs to the family of the alphavirus genus *Togaviridae*. It causes a mild illness such as fever and a rash, in immunocompetent individuals.

Period: Emerged in the Americas in 2013 but has been described as early as 1952 in Tanzania.

Epidemiology
It is prevalent in Asia, Africa, Europe, Indian and Pacific infections. The spread of the disease in America originated from the Caribbean. Travel to high-risk areas increases susceptibility to the disease.

Vector
Aedes Aegypti and Aedes Albopictus mosquitoes.

Transmissions
Chikungunya has been identified in 60+ countries throughout Asia, Africa, Europe, North and South America. The virus is transmitted from human to human through the infected mosquito bite.

The virus can be transmitted from the infected

mother to the newborn during birth. However, there is no evidence of the virus transmission through breast milk.

There is a potential for transmission through blood transfusions. No such cases have been reported yet. Once infected, it renders lifelong immunity.

Host
Humans

Incubation Period
Onset of illness occurs between 4-8 days after the bite from an infected mosquito, but symptoms can also be seen as early as 2 days and as late as 12 days after the infected bite.

Clinical Manifestation
Common complaints include fever and joint pain associated with headache, muscle pain, joint swelling, and occasionally a rash. It's not a deadly disease but can exacerbate underlying neurological health issues.

Prevention
An infected person should avoid further mosquito bites during the first week of infection due to the ability to spread the disease to other humans through the infected person's blood via the mosquito vector.
Prevention can be achieved by avoiding mosquito bites. This is done by wearing clothing that covers

arms and legs, using a bug spray with DEET, controlling standing water to keep mosquitoes from laying eggs near water, using mosquito bed nets, and keeping screen doors closed in homes.

TREATMENT

There is no vaccine or cure available at this juncture. Treatment is merely symptomatic including rest, hydration, and acetaminophen as needed for the fever and pain.

Avoid aspirin and Nonsteroidal Anti-Inflammatory Drugs "NSAIDS" i.e., ibuprofen or *Aleve,* until dengue is ruled out as the cause of the disease. NSAIDS and dengue can increase the risk of bleeding.

FAST FACTS

Outbreak: first known in the 1950's Major outbreak in 2013
Origin: Africa (Tanzania) - Asia - South America - Caribbean
Mortality rate: <100,00
Mode of transmission: mosquito
Host: Humans
Symptoms: mostly asymptomatic
Complications: Fever, joint pain
Use DEET, permethrin for prevention - No vaccine - Avoid Travel to endemic areas
Avoid Aspirin and NSAIDS

MALARIA
aka *bad air*

DEFINITION
Malaria emanates from the term *Mal-Aeria* (bad air). It is spread by the bite of an infected mosquito. This is the most common cause of death in the world.

Number of cases: 229 million cases worldwide in 2019.

Number of Deaths: 409,000 deaths worldwide in 2019.

Period: Widely recognized in 4th century B.C however the parasite has been reported to exist for as long as 30 million years. Identification that Malaria was spread by mosquitoes was an important discovery by Major Ronald Ross. While French and other settlers at that time considered *Mal Aer* or bad air to be responsible for the malaria around Panama Canal. The treatment with quinine was also identified at and around the same time.

EPIDEMIOLOGY
Africa, Asia, Caribbean, South Pacific and South America.

Vectors
- Plasmodium Vivax
- Plasmodium Malariae
- Plasmodium Falciparum

Incubation
7-10 days

Clinical Manifestation
- Flu like symptoms
- High grade fever
- Shaking chills

Complications
- Black water fever "Acute Kidney Failure"
- CNS manifestation - seizures, comma, convulsions, meningitis, encephalitis
- Pneumonia

Prophylaxis
- Malarone (Atovaquone/Proguanil)
- One tab once a day
- Start 1-2 days prior to travel
- Continue 7 days after returning

Contraindications
- Pregnant
- Breastfeeding
- Children less than 5 kg

- Patients with kidney disease

CHLOROQUINE
- 300 mg orally/week
- Start 1-2 weeks before trip
- Continue for 4 weeks after returning
- Can be taken in pregnancy
- Can't be used in areas where there is resistance to chloroquine
- Can exacerbate psoriasis
- Not good when not enough lead time before the trip

DOXYCYCLINE
- 100 mg po qd
- Start 1-2 days before the trip
- Continue 4 weeks after returning
- Can't be used in pregnant and children below 8 years
- Least expensive
- Not ideal for short trips
- Avoid sun exposure while taking doxycycline
- Can cause GI upset in some people

MEFLOQUINE
- 250 mg PO Q Daily
- Start 1-2 weeks before trip
- Continue for 4 weeks after returning

- Can exacerbated underlying seizure and psychiatric disorders
- Contraindicated for patients with certain heart conduction abnormalities
- Safe in pregnancy

PRIMAQUINE
- 30 mg PO QD
- One tab once a day
- Start 1-2 days prior to travel
- Continue 7 days after returning
- Can't use in patients with G6PD deficiency
- Contraindicated in pregnancy

TAFENOQUINE
- 200 mg PO QD
- Start 3 days prior to travel
- Continue for 1 week after returning
- Contraindicated in G6PD, pregnant, breast-feeding women and children
- Also, can cause acute psychosis
- Most effective medication for *p-vivax* and *p-falciparum*
- Start 1-2 weeks before travel
- Continue for 4 weeks after returning
- Can be taken in pregnancy
- Cannot be used in areas where there is resistance to chloroquine
- Cannot exacerbate psoriasis

- Not good when not enough lead time before the trip

PREVENTION
- Integrated Mosquito Management
- Aerial spray
- Control of standing water-followed by spray
- DEET
- Mathurin impregnated clothes
- Full sleeve shirts, and long pants

FAST FACTS

Outbreak: ongoing global pandemic
Origin: Africa - Asia - South America - Caribbean
Mortality rate: 5000,00 per year (#1 cause of death in the world)
Mode of transmission: mosquito
Host: Humans
Symptoms: fever, chills, joint pain
Complications: Hepatic Dysfunction, renal failure (black water fever), CNS
Manifestations- seizure, coma, meningitis, encephalitis
Use DEET, permethrin for prevention - No vaccine
Avoid Travel to endemic areas OR take prophylactic medications before travel and continue after returning travelers from the endemic region

WEST NILE DISEASE
WND aka Dead Bird Disease

DEFINITION
Also known as "dead bird disease," this virus spreads through dead birds which have been infected by mosquito bite.

Number of cases: About 40,000 cases have been reported to the CDC since the introduction of the virus to the United States. (Because only a portion of the cases are reported, CDC believes the actual number of cases is around 700,00).

Number of Deaths: >2000 deaths in the US.

Period: First discovered in 1927 in Uganda. First introduced in the US in 1999.

TRANSMISSION
Human transmission occurs through the infected mosquito bite

Human to human transmission
- Infected blood products-transfusion
- Intrauterine-placental transmission
- Through breast milk
- Percutaneous and aerosolized transmission has been described in the laboratory worker

THE NEW PANDEMIC

- Turkey handlers
- Organ donation

Epidemiology
The first reported case was in 1999 in New York, and since has spread to all contiguous states. It was worldwide in 1937. Later WND was responsible for an epidemic and outbreak in the Middle East.

Etiology
Flavivirus

Vectors
Mosquitoes

Host
- Over 300 species of birds have been reported to carry West Nile Virus.
- Scavenger birds such as Crows and jays have been most notorious as a carrier.
- Predatory birds such as Hawks and Owls have also been implicated in the spread of the disease.

Prevention
- Integrated Mosquito Management
- Aerial spray
- Control of standing water-followed by spray
- DEET

CORONAVIRUS AKA COVID-19 - SARS-COV-2

- Mathurin impregnated clothes
- Full sleeve shirts and long pants

CLINICAL MANIFESTATION
Most patients infected with the virus do not exhibit any symptoms.

MILD SYMPTOMS
- Acute febrile illness
- Headaches, body aches
- Nausea, vomiting, diarrhea

SEVERE SYMPTOMS
- >60 years of age and underlying chronic medical conditions
- Meningitis
- Encephalitis
- Flaccid paralysis
- Guillain-Barre Syndrome

DIAGNOSIS
- Antibody IgM-recent infection (positive after once week)
- Antibody IgG-remote infection
- PRNT-plaque-reduction neutralization test
- NAAT-Nucleic Acid Amplification Test from CSF or serum

Treatment

- No vaccine or antiviral available at this juncture.
- Supportive treatment.
- Hospital admission in severe cases.

FAST FACTS

Outbreak: 1927 (Uganda) - 1999 USA
Origin: Africa - North America
Mortality rate: 2000 per year (low mortality)
Mode of transmission: mosquito
Host: Birds "Dead Bird Disease"
Symptoms: fever, chills, joint pain
Complications: CNS manifestations- seizure, coma, meningitis, encephalitis
Use DEET, permethrin for prevention - No vaccine

EASTERN EQUINE ENCEPHALITIS
aka *"EEE" or "arthropod borne viral encephalitis"*

DEFINITION
Severe brain dysfunction which manifests as encephalitis caused by the bite of an infected mosquito.

Number of cases: 107 cases reported 2010-2019 in the US.

Number of Deaths: 48 deaths reported 2010-2019 in the US.

Period: First recognized in horses in the 1830s. First confirmed human case in 1938.

Geography: USA, Europe and Russia

VECTOR
Mosquito
Tick Borne

HOST
Birds - Humans

INCUBATION PERIOD
4-10 days

Clinical Manifestation
Asymptomatic majority of infected patients

Mild symptoms
- Acute febrile illness

Severe symptoms
- Encephalitis
- Meningitis
- Seizures
- Paralysis
- Permanent brain dysfunction

Diagnosis
- PCR from serology from CSF, or brain tissue, in the right clinical context and endemic area.
- EEE-IgM and EEE-IgG.

Treatment
Symptomatic

Mortality
25-30%

Japanese Encephalitis (JE), St. Louis Encephalitis (SLE), Murray Valley Encephalitis (MVE), Venezuelan Equine Encephalitis (VEE) and La Crosse Encephalitis (LCE)

The disease pattern has a similar presentation to the Eastern Equine Encephalitis, with some subtle differences and geographic locations. VEE has the potential to be used as a weapon for bioterrorism and a potential threat to accidental exposure in laboratory workers.

FAST FACTS

Outbreak:
Origin: North America
Mortality rate: few deaths
Mode of transmission: mosquito or tick bite
Host: Infected birds through arthropods
Symptoms: fever, chills, joint pain
Complications: CNS manifestations- seizure, coma, meningitis, encephalitis
Use DEET, permethrin for prevention - No vaccine
Avoid coming in contact with the "dead birds"

ANTHRAX

Definition
Anthrax is a highly infectious disease that can spread to humans by coming in contact with the spores of anthrax either through infected animals in occupational exposure, accidental exposure in the lab or via bioterrorism.

Number of cases: About 2000 cases globally and 5 cases in the US annually.

Number of Deaths: Mortality rates from anthrax vary, depending on exposure. Death results from cutaneous anthrax in approximately 20% of the cases without antibiotics and 25 - 75% for gastrointestinal anthrax; inhalation anthrax has a fatality rate that is 80% or higher.

Period: Clinically described first in 1752 but reported to have originated in 700 B.C

Epidemiology
It's a zoonotic disease that causes herbivorous disease in cattle, sheep, oxen and deer. Anthrax exists round the world in areas where livestock is prevalent like Asia, Africa, Europe and the Americas.

Etiology
Bacillus Anthracis is an anaerobic, gram positive spore encapsulated bacterial spore forming organism which can cause serious illness in both humans and animals.

Transmission
- Usually not contagious.
- Human to human transmission may occur if an infected person comes into contact with a person with skin ulcers or tears.
- Spores of *B Anthracis* gain access via multiple routes.

Inhalational
- Industrial-animal workers
- Bioterrorism

Food sources
- Contaminated food i.e. consuming infected, undercooked animal meat. It is less
- Common in the USA during USDA strict regulatory compliance with animals
- Vaccination and enforced guidelines for slaughterhouses
- Contaminated potable water sources
- Entry through the skin or soft tissue when the architectural integrity is
- compromised i.e., any ulcers or skin breakdown

Human to Human transmission-rare
Zoonotic transmission from animals i.e., sheep to humans, like sheep and animal handlers who come in contact with an infected animal in a slaughterhouse. Also called *"Wool sorters Disease."*

Bio-weapon-Bioterrorism
- Mail delivery-powdered form
- Aerosolization route
- Contamination of the water source

Injection anthrax-by heroin or IV drug users

Epidemiology
Robert Koch was the first scientist to report Anthrax as a microbe during the late 1800's. Louis Pasteur developed an anthrax vaccine in 1881. However, before this, Anthrax was a common occurrence in the annals of history. It was thought to have been mentioned in 700 BC, where herds of horses, sheep, camels and cattle were infected and died in great numbers. It was also prevalent in Egypt and Mesopotamia, with an honorable mention in the Book of Genesis.

Clinical Manifestation

Constitutional symptoms
- Fever
- Myalgia

Classification-Types of Anthrax

Cutaneous-Dermatologic Anthrax
- 95-99% of cases.
- Itchy skin blisters.

- Painless skin ulcers on exposed surfaces, i.e., hands, neck, face.

Inhalation-Pulmonary Anthrax (most serious and deadly form)
- Cough
- Shortness of breath
- Sore throat
- Chest pain
- Swelling of neck or lymph nodes
- Respiratory failure
- Sepsis syndrome

Gastrointestinal Anthrax
- Nausea, vomiting, diarrhea
- Difficulty swallowing - dysphagia
- Abdominal pain and swelling

Anthrax Meningitis
- Host of neurological presentations.

Injection Anthrax
- This is a local skin and soft tissue reaction to anthrax injection, which is usually due to an accidental injection or is intentional.
- Administered to induce antibody responses, i.e., selected military and healthcare workers.
- Fever and chills.
- Pain at the site of infection.

- Localized blister formation with black center.
- Occasional induration, swelling of the skin underlying soft tissue and muscles.
- Localized abscess formation may occur.

Diagnosis

A quick and reliable diagnosis can be obtained through a centralized lab, i.e., Laboratory Response Network or LRN. This lab was set up in collaboration with the FBI, CDC and Association of Public Health Lab (APHL).

PCR of Sputum, CSF or wound specimens can be sent for local surveillance testing of *Bacillus Anthracis*, which is followed by confirmatory testing at the central labs.

Treatment

Vaccine
Usually dispensed to the military personnel

Antibiotics
- Fluoroquinolones-Ciprofloxacin
- Doxycycline
- Vancomycin
- Carbapenems
- Single, combination oral and IV medication can be used depending on severity, presentation and clinical indication.

Antitoxins
- ABthrax
- Anthrasil

Combination of antimicrobial-antitoxin therapy was found to be superior to use of either agent when administered alone. Especially when there is a late presentation beyond 60 hours.

Hospitalization and aggressive critical care management may be needed in some severe cases.

FATALITY RATE
- 90-100%, without treatment (almost fatal without treatment).
- 50% with treatment.

FAST FACTS

Outbreak: Reported in the BC era, most recent in 1800's
Origin: unknown
Mortality rate: few deaths
Mode of transmission: animals, lab exposure, bioterrorism
Host: Infected animals
Symptoms: respiratory, GI or skin
Complications: pneumonia "widened mediastinum" CXR
Treatment: Highly treatable with antibiotics when initiated early - antitoxins

PLAGUE
aka BLACK DEATH

DEFINITION
Plague is a disease that affects humans and other mammals. It is caused by the bacterium, *Yersinia pestis*. Humans usually contract plague after being bitten by a rodent flea that is carrying the plague bacterium or by handling an animal infected with the plague.

Number of cases: Worldwide, there were 3,248 cases reported from 2010 to 2015.

Worldwide - 1,000 to 2,000 cases are reported to the WHO each year.

United States - 1,006 confirmed/possible plague cases from introduction year of 1900-2012

- 80% of plague cases in the US have been bubonic plagues.

Number of Deaths: 584 deaths worldwide from 2010 to 2015.

Death Rate Before antibiotics, from 1900-1941 the mortality rate was 66% in the United States. After antibiotics, the mortality rate has been lowered to about 11%.

Period: Incubation period of 3-7 days.

Etiology
It is caused by a bacterium called *Yersinia Pestis*.

Transmission
- Flea bites
- Through infected rodents when they come in contact with humans and other mammals.
- Dogs and cats can also bring it home when they come in contact with infected rodents.
- Inhalation

Vector
Fleas

Epidemiology
The plague got its notoriety during the medieval period. Along with great death and destruction, the Plague had such a cultural impact that religious communities like the Jews were blamed for the illness during the Black Death pandemic of 1348-1351. Many Jews were killed senselessly. If one had contracted the Black Death, they were thought to have incurred the wrath of God for being sinful. Things are certainly better today but scapegoating sadly still exists. Plague is an example of a recurrent pandemic, as it impacted Asia and Europe multiple times. Resulting the loss of major human life and livestock, the plague still returns

in small waves in some parts of Africa, Asia and the Americas. Yersinia circulates between mammals and its flea vectors at a slower rate, therefore serving as a long-term reservoir. The western half of the USA has some plague endemic areas. A majority of United States cases are that of the bubonic type. Less than 20 cases of plague are reported each year across the contiguous United States. There is no gender or age predilection, as women and men from infancy to geriatric age groups are affected. Men slightly have increased risk due to engagement in outdoor activity.

Constitutional Symptoms
- Fevers
- Chills
- Myalgias

BUBONIC PLAGUE

The most common manifestation of the Plague, the Bubonic Plague shows itself through enlarged lymph nodes on the face, neck, axilla and groin, called "buboes." These painful, but not fluctuant sores are formed by infection and inflammation of lymph nodes.

SEPTICEMIC PLAGUE

Like the bubonic plague, the Septicemic Plague presents with sepsis, when one is exposed to infected body fluids or tissues. A common occurrence among hunters when skinning an infected animal. It can present through septic shock.

PNEUMONIC PLAGUE
This form of plague is contracted by the inhalation of infectious droplets, containing plague bacteria. Presents as pneumonia or symptoms of respiratory tract infection, shortness of breath, cough and chest pain. This is the highest contagious disease as it can be spread from humans to humans. Mortality with this form of plague reaches 100%.

YERSINIA ENTEROCOLITICA
This is a bacterium that is most commonly spread through the consumption of raw or uncooked pork, however, other animals such as cattle and rodents can also carry this strain. Fever, diarrhea, and abdominal pain are common symptoms in children while abdominal pain and fever are the more dominant symptoms in adults.

DIAGNOSIS
- Travel to endemic areas, with appropriate symptoms of sudden onset of fever and lymphadenopathy
- Isolation of the organism in culture obtained from serum and sampling of the lymph nodes.

Treatment
7-14 days of;
- Streptomycin
- Gentamicin
- Doxycycline
- Tetracycline
- Fluoroquinolones are also one of the alternatives

Prevention
- Rodent prevention.
- Wearing protective gloves when handling animals in the endemic are the Flea mitigation strategies, including repellent sprays, DEET, and permethrin.
- Infected clothing.
- Keep pets safe from infected fleas.
- Don't allow outdoor pets in endemic areas to sleep in your beds.

PUI's-Person Under Investigation
- Place in strict contact and droplet isolation, unless either testing or pneumonia or skin lesions have been ruled out.
- 48 hours of appropriate antibiotics should be administered before isolation is discontinued.

Post Exposure Prophylaxis
- Doxycycline 100 mg orally once a day for seven days.

- Bactrim can be used in pregnant women and children.
- Any person who comes in contact with, face to face or within 3 feet of known or suspected disease.

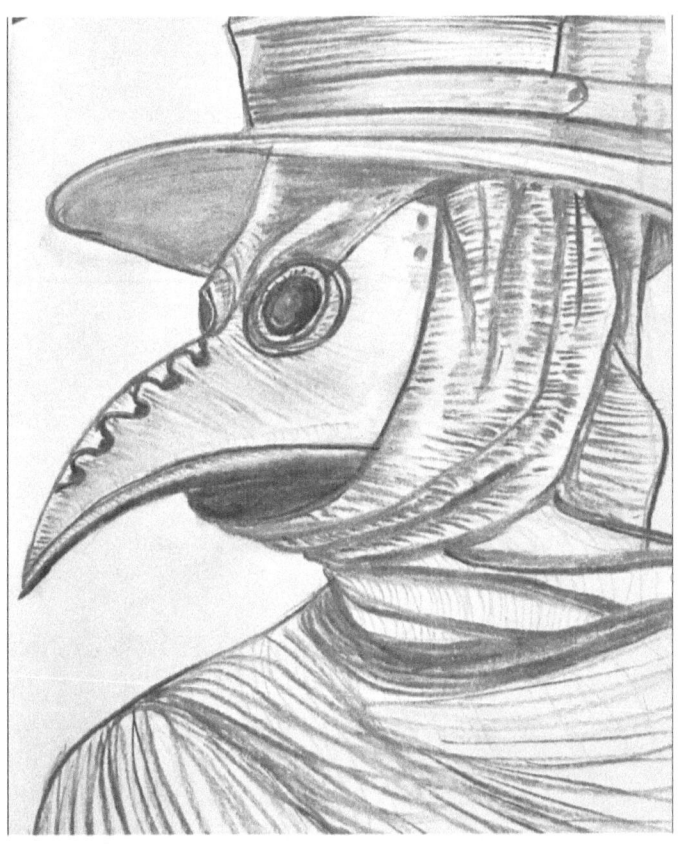

"Plague Doctors' Mask" by *Khalida Anwar, MD*

THE NEW PANDEMIC

> **FAST FACTS**
>
> Outbreak: 1346-1353
> Origin: Africa and Eurasia
> Mortality: 75-200 million deaths during the outbreak of 1346
> Mode of transmission: Fleas - rodents - cats - lab accident
> Host: Infected fleas
> Symptoms: skin, respiratory manifestations or septicemia
> Complications: buboes (enlarged lymph nodes), pneumonia respiratory failure
> Treatment: Tetra - doxycycline

SMALLPOX

DEFINITION
Smallpox is an infectious disease caused by the Variola virus.

Period: The last natural outbreak in the United States was in 1949.

EPIDEMIOLOGY
The disease has been eradicated from the USA since 1978, when the last person from smallpox died. Last major outbreak in the USA was in the 40's. First instance of smallpox was reported during the ancient Egyptian era, as there is evidence of smallpox in *Ramses' mummy*. Smallpox pandemic was responsible for annihilation of the Aztecs and South American Native populace after Spanish incursion and massacre. Nearly 90% of the local population perished as either a direct result of the infection and its sequelae or a resultant hunger, as there was no one left to take care of the sick. There were various religious connotations to the disease as it held its grip across the globe. Various celestial deities, worship and dances were associated with the disease.

ETIOLOGY
Variola Virus

Transmission

Although smallpox is now eradicated, it used to spread from human to human. Smallpox could spread as early as the presence of the first sores on an infected person's mouth or throat. Smallpox spreads via droplets from an infected person's mouth, nose, or through cough. Additionally, the scabs were filled the fluid containing the variola virus would spread through direct contact of objects touched by an infected person like clothing.

Vaccine

The Smallpox vaccine emanated from the ancient practice of variolation. The process by which substances form the pustules of patients with the milder diseases, called "variola minor" to inoculate healthy individuals. This phenomenon was first practiced by Dr. Jenner in the early 1800's. However, similar records of vaccination have been reported in Chinese literature during the Ming Dynasty, when the powdered pus was inoculated in the nose of healthy people to attain immunity.

Incubation Period

Anythefrom 7-19 days.

Clinical Manifestation

Early Symptoms include
- Fever >101'F
- Headaches
- Body Aches

CORONAVIRUS AKA COVID-19 - SARS-COV-2

- Nausea and Vomiting
- Early rash would present around day 4 with thick opaque filled skin sores with a dented center.
- Around day 6 of infection, lasting for roughly 10 days. The rash turns into infectious pustules which are rounded, sharply raised, and firm to the touch. After about 5 days then the rash would crust over with scabs formation.
- After roughly 3 weeks the scabs would fall off leaving scar-like marks on the skin The patient is still contagious until the last scab is gone.

MORTALITY
30%
Survivors were left with permanent scars and blindness.

FAST FACTS

Outbreak: 1949 -Eradicated in the USA since 1970'S
Origin: Africa - Asia
South American population was devastated after Spanish Inquisition
Mortality rate: few deaths
Mode of transmission: humans - humans via coming in contact with droplet, skin or secretions
Host: humans
Symptoms: fever, chills, joint pain
Complications: pneumonia, neurologic manifestation, blindness
vaccine available

MONKEYPOX

DEFINITION
A rare viral disease caused by the monkeypox virus, *Orthopoxvirus poxviridae*. Monkeypox is found in Central and Western Africa but has been documented outside of Africa in the United States, United Kingdom, and Israel.

Number of cases: >1369 since 1970 with >1000 cases in Congo. 47 cases in the United States in 2003.

Number of Deaths: In Africa, the case fatality rate is 1-15% with the highest risk of death being in young children.

Period: Monkey Pox was first discovered in 1958 when the first two outbreaks were identified in monkey colonies. The first human case was recorded in 1970.

Closely resembles that of smallpox infection, except that monkeypox presents with lymphadenopathy. This can be generalized or localized i.e., face or armpits-axilla, or can have diffused and systemic presentation. There is also travel history to endemic areas i.e., Central and West Africa.

EPIDEMIOLOGY
Monkeypox has been reported in humans in central and West-African countries. Human monkeypox

infections have only been documented three times outside of Africa; in the United States in 2003 (47 cases), and in both the United Kingdom (3 cases) and Israel (1 case) in 2018.

Etiology
Monkeypox virus, *Orthopoxvirus poxviridae*.

Transmission
The transmission of monkeypox can be through respiratory droplets or through infected fluids or lesions. Monkeypox can enter the body through the respiratory tract, broken skin, or mucous membranes after a person comes in contact with an infected person, animal, or material.

Incubation Period
5-21 days, but typically 7-14 days.

Clinical Manifestation
Early symptoms include fever, headache, muscle aches, back ache, swollen lymph nodes and chills.

Within 1-3 days the patient typically starts to develop a fever and a rash that begins on the face and spreads to the rest of the body.

The lesions progress from macules to papules to vesicles to pustules to scabs before the fall off around 4 weeks from the start of the infection.

FAST FACTS

Outbreak: USA, UK, Israel, Africa
Origin: Africa in 1958
Mortality rate: few deaths
Mode of transmission: humans - humans via coming in contact with droplet, skin
or secretions
Host: humans
Symptoms: rash, fever, chills, joint pain
Complications: pneumonia, neurologic manifestation

CHICKEN POX
aka Varicella

DEFINITION
An acute and highly contagious disease, which is caused by varicella Zoster Virus-VZV. VZV is a DNA virus, a member of the herpesvirus group. Once a person is infected with VZV, it tends to stay as a latent virus in the neuronal ganglia/tissues and can get reactivated once the immune system is compromised presenting as *Shingles*.

Number of cases: 4 million cases in 1972, 15,427 cases in 2010 and 8,775 cases in 2017.

Number of Deaths: 100 deaths in 1972, 4 in 2010 and 2 in 2017.

Period: 1767 to present.

EPIDEMIOLOGY
Originated in Africa millions of years ago. First Differentiated from smallpox and defined in 1767. In 1875, high contagiousness was documented. The first association between shingles and chickenpox was made in 1888. In 1954, varicella virus was isolated from both chickenpox and shingles lesions. Chickenpox became nationally notifiable in 1972. Nearly 4 million infections occurred each year at that time

resulting in 100 deaths and 10,000 hospitalizations. In 1994-1995, the chickenpox vaccine was licensed. Gradually vaccine usage increased among the general population. In 2010, 15,427 cases were reported with 4 deaths. In 2017, 8,775 cases were reported with 2 deaths.

Transmission
- Human to Human via close contact.
- Highly contagious.
- Aerosolization.
- Infected respiratory secretions.

Incubation Period
10-20 days

Clinical Manifestation
The symptoms usually manifest in children as 200-500 small itchy, blistery rashes on the face and trunk and spread to the rest of the body. This is a highly contagious viral disease which can be quite deadly in children, adolescents, pregnant and immunocompromised individuals i.e., HIV/AIDS and patients with malignancy or on chemotherapeutic agents.

Diagnosis
Clinical presentation with rash in an unvaccinated child or immunocompromised individual.

Constitutional-Generalized Features
- Fever
- Malaise
- Headache
- Loss of appetite

Specific Features
- Maculo-papular or vesicular itchy, blistery rash, lasting 4-7 days.
- These rashes ultimately turn into scabs and are present in all stages of development.

Complications
- Pneumonia
- Sepsis
- Encephalitis
- Skin infections-necrotizing fasciitis
- Dehydration
- Toxic shock syndrome
- Osteomyelitis
- Septic arthritis

Shingles
- Reactivation of the prior chicken pox or varicella in unvaccinated adults.
- Patient is contagious 1-2 days prior to the onset of symptoms, until all rashes have turned into scabs.
- Vaccinated people who end up getting a rash

usually don't scab. These individuals are considered non-contagious once there is no new crop of skin lesions or rashes.

TREATMENT
- Isolate the infected person.
- Hydrate.
- Calamine lotion to prevent itching and hence secondary skin infections as the rash is very itchy.
- Cool baths with baking soda.
- Uncooked oatmeal for the itching.
- Trim fingernails.
- Mittens.
- Avoid using aspirin in children, as they can develop Reye's Syndrome-use acetaminophen instead.
- Antiviral Therapy
  - Acyclovir-oral or IV
  - Valacyclovir
  - Famciclovir
  - Foscarnet
- Antibiotics for the secondary infections, i.e., pneumonia, skin infections or CNS infections.

HOSPITAL/FACILITY MANAGEMENT
- Negative pressure-isolation room.
- Contact and Airborne isolation until lesions are all crusted.

- No contact with visitors who are not immunized.
- Only immunized healthcare should be allowed to provide direct care of the patient.

VACCINATION
- Varicella vaccine is readily available and can prevent morbidity and mortality associated with the disease.
- Vaccinated individuals are still contagious.
- Two doses are recommended.

FAST FACTS
Outbreak: 1970's - 2010 - 2017
Origin: Africa - Asia 1767
Mortality rate: few deaths
Mode of transmission: humans - humans via coming in contact with droplet, skin or secretions
Host: humans - "Chickenpox in children" and "Shingles in adults"
Symptoms: rash, fever, chills, joint pain
Complications: pneumonia, neurologic manifestation vaccine available for children and adults

POLIO - POLIOMYELITIS

Definition
An acute viral disease, transmitted via an oral-fecal route through "poor hygiene practices" and is caused by the *poliovirus*.

Number of cases: 42 cases of paralytic polio reported in 2016 (Note that only 0.5% of the people infected with polio develop paralytic polio).

Number of Deaths: No deaths reported in the past decade in the US. However, during its peak in the 1940s, it afflicted 35,000 people per year.

Period: Existed as an endemic pathogen for over a thousand years until the 1900s when major epidemics began to occur. It seems to be a major malady in certain parts of the world. In 1934 a significant number of healthcare workers contracted polio virus, i.e., 5% doctors and 11% nurses in LA county. World War II hero and former President Roosevelt is the most famous case of Polio. He was paralyzed and wheelchair bound after contracting the virus, but also was one of the chief advocates of the Polio vaccine. He started the "March of Dimes" which paved the way for widespread vaccination and ultimately the eradication of Polio from the USA in 1979.

Etiology
Human enterovirus with three serotypes.

Epidemiology
A highly infectious disease which is still prevalent in Asia (Pakistan and Afghanistan). Africa declared total eradication of Polio in 2020, while India got rid of it and has been Polio free since 2011. The United States had a major outbreak of polio in the 40's, but it was Polio free by 1979. There has been a resurgence of Polio in Pakistan and Afghanistan. This is because the COVID-19 pandemic has shifted focus away from the problem, and also the strains of Polio have mutated. This is due in part to the thwarting of house-to-house effort to vaccinate children, because of the quarantine. When samples were taken from the sewers there was about a 70% increase in the number of Polio virus strains. Bill and Melinda Gates are major philanthropists behind one of the most expensive campaigns to eradicate viruses by "home to home vaccination program." They have poured in about $17 billion to this campaign so far.

Political Downfall
Multiple political and socioeconomic factors have played a major role in the non-eradication of polio in Afghanistan and Pakistan. Firstly, the Afghan war between the Soviets, and again with U.S troops has limited Polio aid to impoverished areas. People are

THE NEW PANDEMIC

more worried about food and basic human needs as opposed to a Polio vaccine, which they may view as an unnecessary luxury.

The capture of Osama Bin Laden which took place near the Abbottabad province, had undercover western agents posing as Polio medics to gather intel. This has led to a thinking that Polio medics are scouring tribal villages to turn people into the West to kill them, leading to further distrust. In fact, many Polio medics are attacked on site in certain remote tribal areas, especially near the Afghan border. Many are now accompanied by police and paramilitary for protection.

Religious misinformation by militants and hardliner clerics is also playing a major role in the non-vaccination of rural peoples. Many clerics attribute the falling fertility of humans to vaccines, and the Polio and COVID vaccines specifically. Not to mention the fact that anti vaxxer groups in the west are paying these clerics big money to back their anti-vaccination campaigns.

Unfortunately, a lot of this misinformation is spread through Facebook and WhatsApp groups. This is the perfect storm since a lot of tribal peoples save up enough money to buy the newest smartphone, but do not have the education to discern fact from fiction.

Transmission
- Human to human.

- Through feces of the infected person, due to unhygienic practices and contaminated potable water sources.
- Droplets from coughing and sneezing.
- Contaminated toys and objects. Contaminated dirt that children often play with and often put in their mouths seems to be the major route of transmission. Open sewers and gutters often are the major reservoirs of the virus, which often have missing lids, which are sold as scrap metal by the local poor people. The virus travels from mouth to the brain and spinal cord and causes devastating neurological manifestations of disability and consequential devastation and permanent damage if not death.

CLINICAL MANIFESTATION
Constitutional
- Fever
- Sore throat
- Nausea, vomiting and stomach pain

Neurologic
- Acute Flaccid Paralysis
- Post-Polio Syndrome (PPS), a host of neurologic sequelae of muscle weakness
- Paresthesia
- Meningitis

Mortality
2-10%

Vaccine

OPV-oral polio vaccine.

IPV-Inactivated Polio Vaccine.

Administered 2-4-6 months and a booster 4-6 years.

Boosters may be needed one time, if previously vaccinated.

Reports of a mutated form of the virus are resurging, caused by vaccinated children. If unvaccinated people get into contact with the fecal matter of vaccinated people, usually transmitted through open sewers, the conventional vaccine is deemed ineffective. At that point, the virus has mutated and has a new host to replicate further. Therefore, WHO and others are educating people about this common occurrence and are working on developing new vaccines.

Diagnosis

Serology, culture or gene sequencing from the throat, feces, CSF.

Collect two stool specimens 24 hours apart to increase sensitivity.

TREATMENT
- Supportive.
- Ventilatory support if it involves phrenic nerves.
- IVIG has shown some promise albeit no reversal of prior neurologic dysfunction.

FAST FACTS

Outbreak: 1900'S
Origin: Africa - Asia - Europe - USA
Mortality rate: few deaths reported as it has been eradicated except Pakistan and Afghanistan
Mode of transmission: oral-fecal route "poor hygienic conditions"
Host: humans
Symptoms: acute diarrheal illness
Complications: neurologic manifestation, paralysis, post-polio syndrome
vaccine widely available

MEASLES

Definition
This is an acute upper respiratory viral illness caused by morbillivirus of the paramyxoviridae family.

Number of cases: 1282 cases in 2019 (highest since 1992) in the US. Globally about 10 million people are infected each year.

Number of Deaths: 91,000 deaths every year globally.

Period: 7th century A.D. to Present.

Etiology
Measles virus is a single stranded, enveloped virus with only one serotype.

It belongs to the morbillivirus of the paramyxoviridae family.

Epidemiology
Since the turn of the century, 2000 the measles has been eliminated from the USA. About 10 million people are affected by measles each year. There are occasional outbreaks in the USA, which are related areas where unvaccinated immigrants arrive or groups of anti-vaxxers. It is still prevalent in Asia, Africa and South America.

Transmission
Highly contagious with 90% infectivity.
- Human to human
- Direct contact
- Droplet-remained in the air for 2 hours
- Cough
- Sneezing
- Breathing

Incubation & Infectivity
8 days- 4 days before and 4 days after rash.

Host
Humans are the only known natural host of measles.

Clinical manifestation
- Fever-high grade >105' F
- "3 Cs"
- Cough
- Coryza
- Conjunctivitis
- Kolpik's spot
- Rash
  - Maculopapular.
  - Centrifugal character to the rash as it spreads.

Complications
- SSPE- Subacute Sclerosing Panencephalitis- Most deadly complication.
- Diarrhea
- Pneumonia
- Otitis media

Diagnosis
Serum, urine and respiratory secretion test.
- IgM
- RT-PCR
- Genotyping

Vaccine
- MMR-Measles Mumps and Rubella.
- MMRV-Measles Mumps Rubella and Varicella.
- 2 doses are recommended in children and un-vaccinated post high school students.
- A single dose of MMR is recommended in adults who were never vaccinated.

Contra-indication to vaccine
- Pregnant.
- Immune compromised.
- TB
- Allergies to any of its components.
- Any other vaccination within the past 4 weeks.

Post Exposure Prophylaxis
- MMR vaccine
- IGIM - Intramuscular Immunoglobulin G

Treatment
- There is no specific treatment.
- Symptomatic.
- Vitamin-A supplement.

FAST FACTS

Outbreak: prehistoric
Origin: Africa - Asia
Mortality rate: <100,000 per year
Mode of transmission: humans - humans via coming in contact with droplet, skin or secretions
Host: humans
Symptoms include: "3-Cs" cough, coryza, conjunctivitis
Complications: pneumonia, neurologic manifestation
vaccine available

MUMPS

DEFINITION:
Mumps is an infection caused by a paramyxovirus, a member of the Rubivirus family. Also called infectious parotitis, it primarily affects the salivary glands. In childhood, mumps is generally a mild disease, most often affecting children between the ages of five and nine. Adults can be affected with more serious complications.

Number of cases: Prior to 1967, about 186,000 cases were reported yearly, but the actual number of cases were likely much higher due to underreporting. Since the introduction of the 2 dose MMR vaccine in 1989, U.S. mump cases have decreased by 99%. Since 2006 there have been several increases in outbreaks. It is particularly common in close-knit communities and predominantly college-aged students.

Number of Deaths: Deaths from mumps are rare nowadays. There have been no mumps-related deaths reported during recent mumps outbreaks.

Period: Safe and effective vaccines have been available since the 1960s.

Transmission

The mumps virus replicates in the upper respiratory tract. Mumps spreads from human to human via direct contact or by the airborne droplets of a person infected with mumps. The risk of spreading the virus increases the longer and the closer contact a person has with the infected individual.

Incubation Period:

The infectious period is primarily from 2 days before to 5 days after parotitis onset. There have been cases where the virus has been isolated from saliva as early as 7 days prior and 9 days after parotitis occurs. The mumps virus has been isolated for up to 14 days in urine and semen.

Clinical Manifestation

Viral Prodrome
- Flu Like Symptoms.
- Malaise-Fever
- Arthralgia
- Anorexia
- Headaches

Specific Signs and Symptoms
- Parotitis- (swelling of the parotid gland which is different from lymph node swelling).
- Pain, tenderness and swelling of the jaw.
- Ear protrusion.

- Effacement of the jaw angle.
- Severity tends to be less severe in patients with prior vaccination.

Complications
- Permanent deafness
- Encephalitis-meningitis and associated neurological sequelae
- Orchitis-majority is unilateral and hypo fertility and testicular atrophy
- Oophoritis <1% of females
- Mastitis
- Pancreatitis

FAST FACTS

Outbreak: 1967
Origin: unknown
Mortality rate: few deaths
Mode of transmission: humans - humans via coming in contact with droplet, skin or secretions
Host: humans
Symptoms: fever, chills, joint pain "Parotitis"
Complications: pneumonia, neurologic manifestation
MMR vaccine widely available

RUBELLA
aka *"German Measles"*

DEFINITION

Rubella is caused by a virus from the genus *Rubivirus* from the *Togavirus* family (toga means ring). Its symptoms include low-grade fever, respiratory problems, and most notably a rash of pink or light red spots that typically begins on the face and spreads downward, or centrifugally. The rash occurs about two to three weeks after exposure to the virus. In children, illness from rubella infection is usually mild. Complications from rubella are more common in adults than children, and include arthritis, encephalitis, and neuritis.

Virus: *Rubivirus* is an RNA virus which belongs to the *Togavirus*.

Number of cases: About 10 cases annually occurred in the US now. In 1964-1965, there were 12.5 million cases of rubella. Twenty thousand children were born with CRS: 11,000 were deaf, 3,500 blind, and 1,800 mentally disabled.

Number of deaths: In 1964-1965, there were 2,100 neonatal deaths and more than 11,000 abortions – some a spontaneous result of rubella infection in the mother, and others performed surgically after women were informed of the serious risks of rubella exposure during their pregnancy.

Period: First described in 1740. Epidemic in the US 1964-1965.

Clinical Manifestations: Centrifugal rash - starts on the face and spreads to the rest of the body, torso and extremities. Asymptomatic or subclinical infection is also a common form. There is an increased incidence of fetal mortality, morbidity and congenital abnormalities when the infection occurs during pregnancy.

Mode of Transmission: Inhalational or coming in contact with the infectious secretions.

Incubation: Two to three weeks before the classic rash occurs.

Diagnosis: Clinical manifestations or serologic assays.

Treatment: Supportive

Vaccine: One dose of live attenuated vaccine for all after the age of infancy.

CORONAVIRUS AKA COVID-19 - SARS-COV-2

FAST FACTS
Outbreak: 1750 - 1914 -1941
Origin: unknown
Mortality rate: few deaths
Mode of transmission: humans - humans via coming in contact with droplet, skin
or secretions
Host: humans
Symptoms: rash, fever, chills, joint pain "Teratogenic"
Complications: pneumonia, neurologic manifestation
MMR vaccine widely available.

TYPHOID & PARATYPHOID FEVER
aka "Enteric fever"

DEFINITION
An invasive bacterial infection acquired through consumption of contaminated water sources of edible items. The clinical manifestation is a severe episode of acute gastroenteritis.

Number of cases: Worldwide, typhoid fever affects an estimated 11 to 21 million people. In the United States each year, about 350 people are diagnosed with typhoid fever each year.

Number of Deaths: 128,000 and 161,000 deaths every year.

Period: First discovered in 1880. Multiple outbreaks since then.

ETIOLOGY
Salmonella typhi, paratyphoid A, B, C and Salmonella Choleraesuis.

EPIDEMIOLOGY
It is endemic in Southeast and Central Asia.

History
"Typhoid Mary" is a common historical slogan used commonly and pertains loosely to a person carrying transmissible disease. Mary Mallon, an Irish cook (1869-1938), who was an asymptomatic carrier of typhoid was responsible for infecting 58 people with typhoid fever, of whom three succumbed to death. Fun fact, she is also depicted as a supervillain in Marvel comics.

Transmission
Oral fecal route.

Clinical Manifestation
Constitutional
- Fever and chills
- Relative bradycardia
- Salmon colored rash

Gastrointestinal
- Abdominal pain
- Diarrhea
- Intestinal bleeding
- Hepatosplenomegaly
- Peritonitis and perforation may occur.
- Hepatitis

Neurologic
- Sleep related issues.
- Acute psychosis.

- Myelitis.
- Meningitis and encephalopathy.
- Upper motor neuron lesion.
- Stupor, obtundation and comatose status may ensue, bringing in grim prognosis.

Pulmonary

Pneumonia can present in children with acute febrile illness.

Diagnosis
- Travel to endemic areas.
- Anemia, leukopenia-leukocytosis.
- Elevated acute phase reactants, CRP and ESR.
- Abnormal LFTs.
- Widal's Test-limited utility in the endemic area as it can be false positive - in previous infection (tests for antibodies).
- Culture of serum, stool, urine or bone marrow.

Treatment
Medical
Acute Infection
- Azithromycin
- Fluoroquinolones
- Cephalosporin-third generation
- Meropenem-for Extensively Drug Resistant-XDR strains

Chronic Carrier State
- Since they are infectious for prolonged periods >12 months.
- 4 weeks of ciprofloxacin.

Severe Illness
- Dexamethasone 3 mg/kg loading dose followed by 1mg/kg every six hours for 48 hours.

Surgical
If perforation or peritonitis occurs.

VACCINE
Typhoid vaccine is recommended for travel to endemic areas.

FAST FACTS

Outbreak: 1869 Europe
Origin: Africa - Asia (more common in the underdeveloped countries)
Mortality rate: 150,000 deaths per year
Mode of transmission: oral fecal route - consumption of contaminated fluids or
Food - overcrowding
Host: humans - No animal reservoir
Symptoms: gastroenteritis, commonly referred to as "gastro"
Complications: pneumonia, neurologic manifestation
MMR vaccine widely available

NORWALK VIRUS
aka *Cruise Ship Virus - Winter Vomiting Bug*

Definition
A viral disease of the caliciviridae virus that causes an acute onset of gastroenteritis.

Number of cases: 685 million cases worldwide with 200 million cases in children under 5 years old. About 19-21 million cases in the United States.

Number of Deaths: Out of the 19-21 million cases in the United States, 900 people die.

Period: First outbreak identified in 1936. Multiple outbreaks since then mostly on cruise ships.

Epidemiology
Multiple outbreaks have been reported on cruise ships. Outbreaks are reported on a central web-based reporting system called NORS-National outbreak Reporting System.

Etiology
Norovirus belongs to the caliciviridae family of viruses, which is a single stranded RNA virus. There are 33 types of noroviruses that cause gastroenteritis.

Incubation Periods
12-48 hours

Clinical Manifestation
Nausea, vomiting, diarrhea, Low grade fever, myalgia, dehydration and acute renal failure.

Transmission
- Oral-fecal route.
- Contaminated water or ice source.
- Fomites-can survive on clothes and bedsheets for two hours and can survive on surfaces up to 4 weeks.
- Airborne transmission can occur when small particles get airborne during vomiting, coughing or sneezing.
- There is a chance to get it the second time if you get exposed to contaminated food and water.

Diagnosis
- RT-qPCR assay of stool, sputum, vomitus, food and water
- EIA-Enzymatic Induced Immunoassay
- Genotyping

Treatment
- It is a self-limiting disease in the majority of healthy people.

- Symptomatic-fluids-oral or Intravenous - IV.
- No specific treatment or antibiotics-antiviral available.

PREVENTION
- Vigorous and frequent hand washing.
- Cleaning surfaces and making sure water and food sources are clean.
- Lysol and Clorox don't kill norovirus.

FAST FACTS

Outbreak: 1936-multiple associated with cruise ships
Origin: unknown
Mortality rate: < 1000 deaths per year. 20 million affected worldwide-children
Mode of transmission: oral fecal route - consumption of contaminated fluids or
Food - overcrowding
Host: humans - Humans
Symptoms: gastroenteritis, dehydration, electrolyte abnormalities
Complications: shock
Prevention Is the key-aggressive hand hygiene

TUBERCULOSIS - TB

DEFINITION
This is a disease with multiple clinical manifestations which is spread by a bacterium *Mycobacterium Tuberculosis*.

Number of cases: 10 million cases worldwide in 2019. 8,916 cases reported in the United States.

Number of Deaths: 1.4 million deaths worldwide in 2019.

Period: First discovered in 1882.

ETIOLOGY
- *Mycobacterium Tuberculosis*-Pulmonary TB
- *Mycobacterium Leprae*- Leprosy
- *Non-Tuberculosis Mycobacterium - distanet*
- MAC - *Mycobacterium Avium Intracellulare*

EPIDEMIOLOGY
Gained its notoriety from various outbreaks of pulmonary TB at the turn of the century. The number of cases decreased in the Western hemisphere with the advent of reinvigorated public health policies i.e., quarantine (sanatoriums), improved nutritional status and new anti-tuberculosis medication, However, there was a resurgence of the infection after HIV/AIDS became

more common in North America, Europe and Africa. TB still remains endemic in certain geographic regions of Asia and Africa, due to a mere endemic shift. TB has gained a lot of popularity in American culture, and Sanatoriums where TB patients were kept are not famous as hubs for ghost hunting. Sanatoriums were often times unsanitary with unhelpful staff.

TRANSMISSION
- Airborne
- Droplet
- Contact- fomites
- Prolonged exposure in confined spaces.

CLINICAL MANIFESTATION
Constitutional-Generalized
- Low grade fever
- Night sweats
- Weight loss

Pulmonary TB
- Most common presentation
- Chronic cough >3 weeks
- Hemoptysis
- Pneumonia
- Pleural effusion

Extrapulmonary TB
- GI tract

- Cardiac
- Skin
- Kidney
- Spine
- Brain

MDR-TB   Multidrug Resistant

XDR-TB   Extended-Drug Resistant

Latent TB (LTBI)

A form of TB when bacteria can survive in the body without causing overt disease manifestation. LTBI is confirmed by a positive skin test with *Mantoux Test-PPD*. They are neither sick with the disease nor are they contagious. However, they have a predilection to get active TB, if their immune system is compromised.

DIAGNOSIS
Chest X ray.
PPD-*Mantoux Test*.
TB blood testing-IGRA (QuantiFERON Gold)-ideal for patients who had BCG vaccine as a child.
Sputum Acid Fast Bacilli.
Mycobacterial culture.
ADA- Adenosine Deaminase from the pleural or pericardial effusion.

Treatment
General Measure
- Contact, droplet and respiratory isolation.
- Negative Pressure Room.

Medication
- Isoniazid, Rifampin, pyrazinamide, Ethambutol (various combinations).
- Side effects of these medications and combinations need to be monitored.
- Lab testing including CBC, BMP and LFTs should be monitored closely.

Vaccination
- BCG (Bacillus Calmette-Guerin)-administered in children in the TB endemic areas.
  - It is a live-attenuated vaccine.
  - Contraindicated in patients with immunocompromised status.
  - No proven benefits for administering twice in the same individual.
  - New interest in this vaccine as a preventive tool for COVID-19 infection.

Healthcare Workers
- Pre-placement testing for all employees should be done upon hiring.
- Annual testing is not recommended, unless symptomatic or in contact.

- LTBI should be treated in healthcare workers.
  - INH + Rifapentine every week for 3 months.
  - Rifampin every day for 4 months.

Pregnancy
- TB testing and treatment are both recommended during pregnancy.

FAST FACTS

Outbreak: 1892
Origin: Initially was common in Europe - now in Africa - Asia
Mortality rate: 1.4 million deaths per year-10 million cases a year
Mode of transmission: airborne, inhalational, droplet, fomites, overcrowding
Host: humans - Humans
Symptoms include: Respiratory, GI, CNS
Complications: pneumonia, neurologic manifestation
Famous People who died of TB: Eleanor Roosevelt, Thomas Wolf (writer), M Ali Jinnah (politician)

SYPHILIS

Definition
An acute and chronic disease, transmitted through sexual contact, causing the host many manifestations ranging from asymptomatic or otherwise

Number of cases: 30,644 cases reported in the United States in 2017 with 918 cases of congenital syphilis.

Number of Deaths: 64 syphilitic stillbirths and 13 infant deaths in 2017.

Period: First outbreak reported in 1495 with multiple outbreaks since then.

Epidemiology
Syphilis has been around the globe since ancient times. Incidence in the US and worldwide has been decreasing, however. There was a surge in new reported cases in association with HIV, during the 80's and 90's. Speaking of dark science, a study was conducted at Tuskegee by the United States Public Health Services between 1932-1972. This horribly unethical study enrolled around 400 African American males with syphilis. The patients were not treated or told that they were infected with the disease, to study the effects of syphilis on humans. Even though the study lost funding, the study continued. Eventually, 28 patients had

died directly, with one hundred plus died from either complications, or even passed the disease to their children. it was a dark and horribly racist period in American medical science.

ETIOLOGY
Caused by the spirochete *Treponema Pallidum*.

TRANSMISSION
Sexually Transmitted
Vertical transmission
    In utero-from infected mother to the fetus (congenital Syphilis)
    During the birth of a child
Syphilis tends to enhance transmission of HIV/AIDS.

CLASSIFICATION AND CLINICAL MANIFESTATION
    Asymptomatic or Latent Syphilis
    Patients who don't exhibit signs of Syphilis.
- Early Latent
- Symptomatic early stage of the disease.
- Late Latent
- Asymptomatic later stage of the disease.

Classification of Syphilis by chronological staging of the disease

Primary Syphilis
Chancre is a painless localized lesion.

Secondary Syphilis
Diffuse rash.

Tertiary Syphilis
Cardiac disease- Aortic Insufficiency.
Neurosyphilis.
Ocular syphilis - ocular uveitis.

Congenital Syphilis - Vertically transmitted
From infected mother to the child

Diagnosis

Indications for testing
- High risk-symptomatic patient
- HIV/AIDS
- Pregnant
- Sexual partner is diagnosed with Syphilis

Lab Testing

Serologic Testing

Non-treponemal - non-specific - screening
- RPR (Rapid Plasma Reagin)
- VDRL
  Venereal Disease Research Laboratory
- TRUST
  Toluidine Red Unheated Serum Test

Treponemal - specific (antibody testing)
- FTA-ABS
  Fluorescent Treponemal Antibody Absorption Test
- TP-EIA
  Treponema Pallidum-Enzyme Immunoassay
- TPPA
  Treponema Pallidum Particle Agglutination Assay
- CIA
  chemiluminescence immunoassay-one step sandwich assay

TREATMENT
- Penicillin is the drug of choice.
- Ceftriaxone.
- Azithromycin.
- Doxycycline for Penicillin allergy.

NONTREPONEMAL TITERS
These are measured to assess not only reactivity but also the quantities of the antibody. These titers should be obtained prior to initiating therapy and can also be utilized for surveillance and treatment monitoring.

FAST FACTS

Outbreak: 1495 first known, multiple outbreaks since then- Tuskegee Airmen
Origin: Europe - Africa - Asia
Mortality rate: 30,000 annually
Mode of transmission: sexual - AIDS/HIV caused a spike
Host: humans - Humans
Symptoms: skin rash, CNS, cardiac, eye
Complications: pneumonia, neurologic manifestation

RABIES

DEFINITION
Rabies is a neurologic disease caused by a group of neurotropic viruses in the *Rhabdoviridae* species.

Number of cases: In the United States, there has been an average of 2 to 3 reported cases of rabies annually from 1980 to 2015. The true worldwide prevalence of rabies is unknown because of the vast majority of cases occurring in the developing and impoverished world.

Number of Deaths: It is estimated that more than 60,000 people worldwide die of rabies each year and this number is felt to be underestimated.

Period: The average incubation period of rabies is one to three months but can range from several days to years after exposure.

ETIOLOGY
Rabies virus belongs to *Rhabdoviridae* which belongs to *Lyssavirus*.

EPIDEMIOLOGY
About 70,000 worldwide cases of rabies are reported each year. Rabid dogs are responsible for more than 90% of cases. Rabid bats cause the majority

of cases in the USA. Foxes and raccoons are also implicated.

TRANSMISSION
Through the bite of a rabid animal. Once the inoculum is deposited at the skin, the virus travels antegrade through the neuronal axons into the spinal cord and brain. There have been cases of it spreading through aerosolization. Transmission of viruses may also occur with organ transplantation.

FACTORS AFFECTING INFECTIVITY
Genetic susceptibility.
Proximity of the bite to the nervous system.
Size and quantity of the virus inoculum.

INCUBATION PERIOD
1-3 months

CLINICAL MANIFESTATION
Prodrome
- Low grade fever
- Malaise
- Anorexia
- Nausea, vomiting, diarrhea
- Headaches

Localized symptoms - at the site of bite
- Pain

- Paresthesia
- Pruritus

Neurologic Rabies
- Paralytic Rabies
- Encephalitic Rabies
- Hydrophobia
- Seizure

Atypical Rabies
- Associated with rabies caused by bats.
- Neuropathic pain.
- Cranial nerve involvement.
- Choreiform seizure or movement of the involved limb.

Diagnosis
- Skin biopsy.
- Immunofluorescent staining of the skin.
- Isolation of virus from saliva.
- Antibodies to the virus in serum and CSF.

Treatment
- No effective treatment exists.
- Supportive.
- Milwaukee Protocol.
  - Sedation
  - Ventilatory support
  - Anti-seizure medications
  - Avoid steroids

VACCINES
Pre-exposure prophylaxis
- Imovax-rabies vaccine
- Three doses day, 0-7-21

Post Exposure Prophylaxis
- 4 doses, day 0-3-7-14
- Rabies Immune Globulin

FAST FACTS

Outbreak: 1800s
Origin: Africa - Asia - America (bats)
Mortality rate: 60,000 a year
Mode of transmission: bite of the infected animal
Host: dog, bats, racoons, foxes
Symptoms: CNS
Complications: neurologic manifestation, encephalitis, and paralysis
Vaccine: 1885 by Louis Pasteur
People of Southeast Asian descent have a fear of dogs, due to high incidence of rabies in stray dogs in that part of the world. Also, lack of local social practices of keeping a dog as a pet in the household

HEPATITIS A VIRUS (Hep-A)
aka "infectious hepatitis"

DEFINITION
It is an acute infectious disease which can cause a host of GI symptoms, including nausea, vomiting, diarrhea and jaundice. Hep A tends to be endemic in third world countries, due to unhygienic potable water sources and optimal food storage practices.

Number of cases: 32000 in the USA since 2016.

Number of Deaths: >300

Period: 2016-2020

OUTBREAKS
- Frozen strawberries 2016
- Raw Scallops 2016

ETIOLOGIC AGENT
- Hepatitis A Virus-RNA virus

PROPERTIES OF HAV
- Can survive outside humans for months
- Can be killed at 85-degree Celsius for one minute
- Freezing doesn't denature or kill the virus
- Chlorination-kills the virus

Mode of Transmission
- Person to person
- Sexual contact
- Fecal-oral route-drinking, eating contaminated fluids and food.

High Risk Populations
- Gay men
- Travel to an endemic area
- IV drug use
- Exposure to primates
- Household contact
- Patient with bleeding-coagulation disorder

Incubation Period
- 15-50 (average one month)
- Resolves in 2-6 months

Clinical Manifestation
- Self-limiting disease
- Fever
- Headaches
- Anorexia
- Nausea, vomiting, diarrhea
- Jaundice
- Abnormal LFTs
- Clay colored stool
- Dark urine

Vaccination
- HAVRIX
- VAQTA
- TWINRIX
- IgG-GamaStan
- Hepatitis A Vaccine- 2 doses can be given to age 1 years and greater.
- Antibodies produced as a result of infection or vaccination confer life-long immunity-can't get re-infected.
- Pre-vaccination serology is not required prior to giving the vaccine.

Vaccination Contraindication
- Allergy to one of its components
- Patient who is sick
- Safe in pregnancy and HIV

Diagnosis
IgM to anti HAV
PCR or genotyping for HAV antigen

Treatment
- No specific treatment is available
- Supportive, fluid resuscitation and electrolyte replacement either PO or IV
- Post exposure prophylaxis
- Rigorous hygiene techniques

FAST FACTS

Outbreak: Multiple
Origin: Africa - Asia
Mortality rate: very low <1%
Mode of transmission: fecal-oral route
Host: humans - Humans
Symptoms: GI, liver "Jaundice-self-limiting disease
Complications: acute fulminant hepatic failure
Vaccine: Get vaccinated when travelling to third world countries, Asia, Africa

HEPATITIS B VIRUS (HBV)

Definition
It is a chronic liver infection caused by Hepatitis B Virus. This virus is transmitted by blood, blood transfusions, bodily fluids or sexual transmission. Needle stick is one of the common modes of transmission especially amongst healthcare workers.

Number of cases: 250 million carriers worldwide

Number of Deaths: 600,000 per year

Period: First discovered in 1965.

Etiology
HBV-is a double stranded DNA Virus, which belongs to the hepadnavirus family of viruses.

Mode of transmission
- Sexual transmission, heterosexual and homosexual.
- IV drug abuse.
- Iatrogenic-surgery, central line placement or IV access.
- Transplacental to the fetus (vertical transmission).
- Sharing razors, toothbrush and glucose monitoring equipment and needles.
- Any blood or blood product could be potentially infectious, even dried up, can be infectious.

- Transplantation of organs infected with HBV.

INCUBATION PERIOD
3 months

PROPERTIES OF HBV
HBV can survive outside the body for 7 days, hence universal precaution should be exercised even when handling dried up blood or blood products.

HIGH RISK POPULATION
- Healthcare workers
- Cancer chemotherapy
  - Rituximab
- Immune Modulating drugs
  - TNF alpha Inhibitor
  - Chronic high dose steroids
- Organ transplantation and anti-rejection medications.
- Patient being treated for Hepatitis C.
- Homosexuality is higher risk, but transmission can occur heterosexually when proper barrier methods of contraception are not used.
- Travel to endemic areas predisposes especially to high-risk individuals.
- IV drug use when sharing the contaminated needles.
- Exposure to primates.
- Household contact.
- Patient with bleeding-coagulation disorder.

Degree-Duration of Illness
Childhood disease   90% result in carrier state
Adulthood disease   2-6% result in carrier state

Clinical Manifestations

Acute Hepatitis B
- Most patients may be asymptomatic or remain as carriers.
- Fulminant Hepatitis is the most detrimental outcome of the disease.
- Fever, malaise.
- Headaches.
- Anorexia.
- Nausea, vomiting, diarrhea.
- Jaundice.
- Abnormal liver function tests.
- Clay colored stools
- Dark urine.

Chronic Hepatitis B (HBsAg >6 months)
- Liver cirrhosis occurs when a patient is untreated for prolonged periods of time.
- Hepatocellular Carcinoma can occur in patients with chronic long-standing cirrhosis.

Diagnosis
Serology
   Antigen testing
   - HB-sAg

- HB-cAg
- HB-eAg

Antibody testing
- Ig-M (recent infection)
- Ig-G (remote infection)

VACCINATION

- Hepatitis B vaccine-series of three injections given at 0-3-6 months.
- Serology should be tested for immune responsiveness, as some people may not mount a good antibody response i.e., non-responders and may require repeated dosing to achieve the optimal antibody titers.
- After vaccination, the surface antibody will be positive for life (HB-surface antibody positive).
- Vaccination can be given to pregnant women, children and immunocompromised individuals.
- Larger and repeat dosing may be needed in a patient with a compromised immune system and on hemodialysis to induce desirable immunity.
- Vaccine can also be administered as a post-exposure prophylaxis, with the first dose given soon after the serology for Hep-B is checked.

There is no added benefit of Hepatitis vaccine in patients who are already infected with HBV

TREATMENT
Acute Infection
- Symptomatic and supportive treatment

Chronic Infection
> Goals of Care
> - Suppression of HBV DNA
> - Loss of HBeAg
> - Loss of HBsAg
> - Individualized approach
> - PEG interferon-*Peg-IFN*
> - Nucleoside-nucleotide analog
>   - Entecavir
>   - Tenofovir

FAST FACTS

Outbreak: Multiple
Origin: unknown 250 million cases worldwide
Mortality rate: 600,000 annually
Mode of transmission: sexual - IV drug users, health care workers, vertical
Transmission from mother to the fetus
Host: humans - Humans
Symptoms: GI - liver "Jaundice
Complications: acute fulminant hepatic failure - chronic carrier state
Vaccine: 3 part series (trilogy) given at 0-3-6 months
Check antibody titres in susceptible individuals
After vaccination "HEP-B-surface antibody" remains positive for life

HEPATITIS C VIRUS (HBC)

Definition
Hepatitis C is an acute or chronic liver infection, which is caused by hepatitis C virus. It is often transmitted through blood or blood products and as a sexually transmitted disease.

Number of cases: 2.4 million people in the US.

Number of Deaths: 8,000-10,000 deaths per year.

Period: Discovered in 1989. Prior to this, it was called non-A non-B hepatitis.

Etiology
HBC-RNA, envelope-shaped virus which belongs to the family of *Flaviviridae*.

Mode of transmission
- Similar to Hep-B virus
- IV drug abuse
- Sexual (more common amongst gay men)
- Iatrogenic
- Organ donation
- Transplacental
- Sharing razors, toothbrush and glucose monitoring equipment and needles

- Blood products even tiny blood, even dried can be infectious
- Tattooing- unregulated

INCUBATION PERIOD
2-12 weeks

PROPERTIES OF HCV
Can survive outside the body.

HIGH RISK POPULATION
- Healthcare workers
- Cancer chemotherapy
  - Rituximab
- Immune Modulating drugs
  - TNF alpha Inhibitor
  - Chronic high dose steroids
- Organ transplantation and anti-rejection medication
- Patient being treated for Hepatitis C
- Homosexuality
- Travel to an endemic area
- IV drug use
- Exposure to primates
- Household contact
- Patient with bleeding-coagulation disorder

DEGREE-DURATION OF ILLNESS
- Acute disease   50%   self-limiting disease

- Chronic disease 50% leads to chronic state and progressive course- HCC, cirrhosis.

CLINICAL MANIFESTATIONS

Acute Hepatitis C
- Most patients may be asymptomatic
- Fever
- Headaches
- Anorexia
- Nausea, vomiting, diarrhea
- Jaundice
- Join pain
- Abnormal Liver function test
- Clay colored stool
- Dark urine

Chronic Hepatitis C
- Liver cirrhosis
- Hepatocellular Carcinoma

Other manifestation of chronic Hep C infection
- Diabetes mellitus
- Kidney Failure due to glomerulonephritis
- Essential mixed cryoglobulinemia
- Porphyria cutanea tarda (Vampire's disease)
- Non-Hodgkin's lymphoma

Diagnosis
- Screening tests for antibodies to HCV (anti-HCV).
  - enzyme immunoassay (EIA)
  - enhanced chemiluminescence immunoassay (CIA)
- Qualitative tests to detect presence or absence of virus (HCV RNA polymerase chain reaction [PCR]).
- Quantitative tests to detect the amount (titer) of virus (HCV RNA PCR).

Vaccination
There is no vaccination available.

Genotypes
- There are 67 genotypes of Hep C virus.
- Type 1 is most common in the US - 70% of cases.

Treatment
- Referral to a hepatologist, GI, ID, Internist.
- Liver function test.
- Genotyping.
- Check HIV status.
- Check for other hepatitides.

Specific Treatments

There are multiple oral combination therapies available for eradication of the virus, with *Harvoni* leading the group.

FAST FACTS

Outbreak: Multiple
Origin: unknown
Mortality rate: 600,000 annually
Mode of transmission: sexual - IV drug users, health care workers, vertical
Transmission from mother to the fetus
Host: humans - Humans
Symptoms: GI - liver
Complications: acute fulminant hepatic failure - chronic carrier state

HEPATITIS D VIRUS
aka "Delta Hepatitis" or HDV

DEFINITION
This is another form of hepatitis which is caused by hepatitis D virus (HDV). Hepatitis D can only occur in patients who are already infected with hepatitis B virus.

Number of cases: No official surveillance in the US, because of the low number of cases. About 5% of the cases of chronic hepatitis B can develop a hepatitis D superinfection.

Number of Deaths: Case fatality rate of about 20%

Period: Discovered in 1977

ETIOLOGY
Hepatitis D Virus is an incomplete RNA virus which needs co-infection with Hepatitis B to produce infectivity.

EPIDEMIOLOGY
A few cases are present in the USA, mostly from immigrants from the endemic arrears which are co-infected with HBV. DHV is endemic in Europe, Mediterranean, Asia, Africa and South America.

GENOTYPES
There are eight genotypes, which are widespread across the globe.

INCUBATION PERIOD
3-7 weeks

MODE OF TRANSMISSION
- IV drug abuse.
- Sexual (more common in homosexual men).
- Iatrogenic.
- Organ donation.
- Transplacental transmission is rare.
- Sharing razors, toothbrush and glucose monitoring equipment and needles.
- Blood products, even tiny blood, even dried can be infectious.

HIGH RISK POPULATIONS
- Healthcare workers
- Cancer chemotherapy
    - Rituximab
- Immune Modulating drugs
    - TNF alpha Inhibitor
    - Chronic high dose steroids
- Organ transplantation and anti-rejection medication
- Patient being treated for Hepatitis C
- Homosexual men

- Travel to an endemic area
- IV drug use
- Exposure to primates
- Household contact
- Patient with bleeding-coagulation disorder

CLINICAL MANIFESTATIONS
Acute Hepatitis D/B Co-infection
- Most patients may be asymptomatic   95%
- Fulminant Hepatitis   5%
- Fever
- Headaches
- Anorexia
- Nausea, vomiting, diarrhea
- Jaundice
- Abnormal Liver function test
- Clay colored stool
- Dark urine

Chronic Hepatitis D Superinfection
- Accelerates the progressions of HPV by 70-90-%
- Liver cirrhosis
- Hepatocellular Carcinoma

DIAGNOSIS
Serology confirming the presence of HDV antibodies or detection of HDV-RNA.

Every person infected with HBV should be screened for it, especially those at high risk and from the endemic area.

Treatment
- No specific treatment modality is available.
- Treatment with *Pegylated Interferon Alpha* initially showed some response, but persistent efficacy only showed subtle improvement, therefore not widely used.
- Liver transplantation is the only viable option, especially when a fulminant course ensues.

Vaccination
- No vaccine has yet been developed.
- However, HBV vaccine is recommended in high-risk patients to mitigate sequelae of co-infection with HBV.

FAST FACTS

Outbreak: less common
Origin: unknown
Mortality rate: low - defective virus - requires co-infection with Hep B
Mode of transmission: sexual - IV drug users, health care workers, vertical
Transmission from mother to the fetus
Host: humans - Humans
Symptoms: GI - liver "Jaundice
Complications: acute fulminant hepatic failure - chronic carrier state

HEPATITIS E VIRUS
aka "HEV"

DEFINITION
An acute liver disease caused by hepatitis E virus. It is usually caused by contracting the virus in the endemic area or a disaster zone, by drinking contaminated water or food. This is a self-limiting disease and is not transmitted sexually.

Number of cases: No official surveillance in the US, because of the low number of cases. About 20 million infections worldwide with about 3.3 million cases that become symptomatic.

Number of Deaths: About 44,000 deaths in 2015.

Period: First discovered in 1983.

ETIOLOGY
Hepatitis E Virus is a single stranded virus which belongs to the Herpesviridae family.

EPIDEMIOLOGY
A few cases are present in the USA, mostly from travel from endemic areas, by genotype 3, in men >40 years. It is prevalent in Asia, Africa, the Middle East and South America. Displaced colonies, refugees and communal living increase the risk. It can cause illness

as a sporadic case or as an epidemic, especially after a natural disaster, earthquakes or from wars and political conflicts.

Genotypes
There are four genotypes, which are widespread across the globe.

Incubation Period
15-60 days (40 days average)

Mode of Transmission
- Contaminated water and food sources.
- Fecal-oral route.
- Undercooked and uncooked game meats, venison, wild boar, and pigs.

High Risk Population
Travel in the high-risk area in refugee camps and natural or manmade disaster zones.

Clinical Manifestations
Acute Hepatitis E
- Most patients may be asymptomatic
- Fulminant Hepatitis
- Fever
- Headaches
- Anorexia
- Nausea, vomiting, diarrhea

- Jaundice
- Abnormal Liver function tests.
- Clay colored stool
- Dark urine

Case Fatality Rate
- 1% general population
- 10-30 % in pregnancy (3rd trimester)
- Worst outcomes in patients with underlying chronic liver conditions
- immunosuppression

Chronic Hepatitis E
Chronic disease has not been described with Hepatitis E virus.

Diagnosis
- Serology confirming presence of HEV antibodies or detection of HEV-RNA.
- Especially high risk and travel from the endemic area.

Treatment
- No specific treatment modality is available.
- No specific treatment is available.
- Supportive measures including fluid resuscitation and electrolyte replacement either orally or intravenously.
- Rigorous hygiene techniques.

Prevention
- Hygienic practice, especially when travelling to the endemic areas.
- Boiling-distillation of water or use of iodine tablets.
- Cooking meat properly.
- Avoiding "game meat" in immunocompromised patients.

Vaccination
- No vaccine has been developed.
- However, a recombinant HEV vaccine was approved for use in China.

FAST FACTS

Outbreak: Multiple - 2017 Chad - associated with disaster regions
Origin: unknown - >20 million cases worldwide
Mortality rate: very low <1% - high in pregnancy
Mode of transmission: fecal-oral route, blood and maternal-fetal route
Host: humans - swine - deer, cows, dolphins, primates, bears
Symptoms: GI, liver "Jaundice-self-limiting disease
Complications: acute fulminant hepatic failure

TOXIN MEDIATED DISEASES
Clostridia Species

CLOSTRIDIUM DIFFICILE
aka *"C Diff"*

Definition
This is a gastrointestinal disease caused by toxin producing bacteria which can cause illness ranging from diarrhea to life threatening conditions. It is the most common infectious diarrheal disease in the hospital setting, especially associated with antibiotic use or because of direct contact from the infected patients via healthcare workers or fomites.

Number of cases: >230,000 per year

Number of Deaths: >1200 per year

Period: consistent number of cases and deaths since the advent of modern-day antibiotics.

Classification
- Infectious-active
  - can't survive in the environment for prolonged periods.
- Non-infectious
  - Spores-can stay dormant for prolonged periods.

- Pans, stethoscopes, neck ties, rings, phones have been implicated.

PATHOGENESIS

The clostridium difficile spores can hide in the colon for a prolonged period. Once the normal defense mechanism which is guarded by the colonic commensal is compromised or altered, especially after antibiotic use, the C-diff spores germinate and degranulate to become an active, infectious bacteria, causing havoc. As a result, toxins are released causing pseudomembranous colitis which result in diarrheal manifestation along with the systemic sequelae.

PREDISPOSITION

Antibiotics
- Clindamycin (most notorious)
- Penicillin's
- Cephalosporins

MEDICAL CONDITIONS

Ulcerative Colitis can predispose without antibiotics.

CLINICAL MANIFESTATION

- Abdominal pain
- Nausea, vomiting
- Diarrhea
- Fever
- Sepsis

- Shock
- Dehydration
- Toxic Megacolon - most feared and often fatal complication

ETIOLOGY
- It is usually caused in association with the use of antibiotics
- Age >65 years
- Immunocompromised
- Hospitalized
- Nursing home resident
- Nurseries

TRANSMISSIBILITY
- Person to person
- Contact with soiled linen or fomites

DIAGNOSIS
- *C-diff* toxins from stool specimens
- Elevated WBC count

TREATMENT
- Flagyl - oral or IV.
- Vancomycin is recommended as a first line regimen in patients with severe c diff infection.
- Supportive management- fluid and electrolyte balance.
- Stool transplantation - resistant cases.

THE NEW PANDEMIC

> **FAST FACTS**
>
> Outbreak: Multiple associated with the use of antibiotics - healthcare setting
> Most common nosocomial infection (healthcare acquired)
> Origin: unknown - more common in the developed countries
> Mortality rate: varies
> Mode of transmission: spores, contact
> Host: humans - Humans
> Symptoms: diarrhea, fluid and electrolyte imbalance, shock
> Complications: chronic carrier state, toxic megacolon

CLOSTRIDIUM TETANI
aka "Lockjaw" or " stiff person syndrome"

DEFINITION
This disease is caused by a rod shaped, spore forming bacterium which is often found in the soil and intestines. It manifests as spasmodic contraction of the muscle, most commonly jaw muscles. It remains dormant in the soil as a spore, it penetrates and accesses humans and animals. It has an exotoxin which can cause severe spasms upon muscle penetration. When muscles of the neck and jaw become spasmodic, it can result in a condition called "lockjaw" or *tetani*.

Number of cases: 30 reported cases a year.

Number of Deaths: Mortality is high when the disease sets in. There have been only 19 deaths reported out of 30 cases reported in a decade between 2008-2018.

Period: First reported in 1889 by Kitasato Shibasaburo.

TRANSMISSION
There is no human-to-human transmission. Through spores, which are present in the soil, dust and manure can penetrate skin through any break in the skin, or existing wound and germinate, releasing the exotoxin.

Incubation Period
3-21 days, averaging about 10 days

Clinical Manifestations
- Muscle spasm, i.e., masseter and neck muscles
- Dysphagia
- laryngospasm
- Seizure
- Headaches
- Lockjaw
- Fractures have been reported
- Aspiration pneumonia

Diagnosis
- Clinical symptoms and signs
- No lab testing available

Treatment
- Supportive and wound care
- Tetanus Immune Globulin (TIG)
- Muscle relaxant
- Paralytics
- Antibiotics
- Tetanus vaccination

Prevention
- Vaccination.
- Tetanus booster every 10 years.

- Good hygiene, including hand washing and wound care.

RISK FACTORS
- Puncture wounds.
- Gunshot wounds.
- Open comminuted and compound fractures.
- Burns.
- IV drug abuse.
- Insect or animal bites.
- Surgical incision site and wounds.

FAST FACTS

Outbreak: not common
Origin: unknown - associated with open contaminated wounds
Mortality rate: low, but is pretty fatal once sets in in unvaccinated people
Mode of transmission: spores, contact
Host: soil - Humans
Symptoms: neurologic, muscle rigidity
Complications: neurologic manifestations
Vaccine widely available

CLOSTRIDIUM BOTULISM
aka Clostridium Botulinum "Botox"

Definition
It is an anaerobic, rod-shaped toxin producing bacterium that is present in the food or honey as a spore. It has gained its notoriety recently due to its cosmetic and medical use for facelifts and treatment of relapsing-remitting migraine.

Number of cases: 182 cases reported in 2017 in the United States.

Number of Deaths: 4 deaths reported in 2017 in the United States.

Period: First discovered in 1735.

Types of Botulinum Toxins
Toxin-A
- This is the agent used for Botox injection.

Toxin-B
- Trade Name *myobloc* is used for the treatment of cervical dystonia. It is used primarily in adults with abnormal neck posturing or dystonia.

Mechanism of Action
Once the toxin accesses the nerve endings, it interferes with the neurotransmitter release, i.e., acetylcholine. This results in the cessation of depolarization, hence muscle paralysis.

Incubation Period
18-36 hours

Clinical Manifestation
- Infants are highly susceptible to toxins in the honey. An array of neurotoxicity is produced.
- Muscle paralysis.
- Respiratory failure if phrenic nerve or diaphragmatic muscles are involved.
- Difficulty swallowing or speaking.
  - Dry mouth.
  - Bilateral facial weakness.
  - Diplopia.
  - Ptosis.
  - Dyspnea.
  - Nausea, vomiting and abdominal cramps.

Epidemiology and Characteristics
Botulinum toxin is one of the most deadly and potent poisons. It has the capacity to kill in very minute quantities i.e., even when less than a millionth of a gram is ingested. The most common and renowned source is home processed canned food and honey, which has

low acid content, i.e., fish, fruits and vegetables. The spores don't survive or thrive in acidic pH i.e., below 4.6. It takes 121-degree Celsius heat for 3 minutes for sterilization, but the process of denaturation occurs at 80 degrees Celsius.

Treatment
- Local wound care if needed.
- Antibiotics
  - Penicillin G
  - Flagyl

FAST FACTS

Outbreak: 1820 - associated with sausage consumption. Also, can occur with canned food and honey (no honey for infants - "BOTOX"
Origin: unknown - more common in the developed countries
Mortality rate: varies
Mode of transmission: spores, ingestion
Host: environment - soil - Humans
Symptoms: diarrhea, fluid and electrolyte imbalance, shock
Complications: life threatening neuroparalysis

CLOSTRIDIUM PERFRINGENS
Aka "Gas Gangrene"

Definition
An anaerobic spore-forming, gram positive bacteria, which can be found in raw meat and poultry. It can use "gas gangrene," when it is able to penetrate skin and soft tissues and has the environment conducive for germination and proliferation. It can also be found in the human intestines.

Number of cases: one million cases a year in the USA.

Number of Deaths: case fatality of < 0.03%

Period: First discovered in 1891.

Pathogenesis
Once gained access via consumption of raw meat, poultry, or other ingestible contaminated sources, it can reach the intestine and release toxins which manifest by an array of host response symptoms including diarrhea.

Epidemiology
One of the spores forming toxin releasing bacteria that can result in "foodborne illness." Cooking at 140 degrees Celsius kills the *C. Perfringens,* development in the vegetative state, but not the endospore

development which can live in the host cell causing disease when there is an opportunity to germinate. Food poisoning can also be caused if the cooked food is not properly stored or preserved. It can also be present in soups, sauces and gravy. Spores are readily found in feces, soil, air and water. *C Perfringens* A is found in the soil and as a normal flora of some animals and also in the human gut. It can also be found inhabiting decaying vegetation and marine sediment.

Host
- Humans
- Dogs

Portal of entry
- GI tract-food poisoning.
- Through wounds or where the integrity of skin is compromised.

Clinical Manifestation
- Abdominal cramps.
- Diarrhea.
- Gas gangrene of *Clostridial* myonecrosis.
- Clostridial necrotizing enteritis.

Incubation Period
6-24 hours after ingesting the contaminated food.

Diagnosis
Inoculate sporulation broth with 1 ml fluid thioglycolate medium culture and incubate 24 h at 35°C. Gram staining of the sporulation broth followed by microscopic examination. *Clostridium perfringens* is a nonmotile anaerobic bacterium.

Treatment
- Supportive.
- Optimal hydration either oral or intravenously.
- Electrolyte replacement.
- Metronidazole, penicillin, macrolides.
- Wound care-debridement as necessary-with myonecrosis.

Prevention
- Since alcohol doesn't kill the spores, handwashing with soap and water is recommended to wash off spores in all spore forming organisms.
- Proper cooking of meat and poultry.
- Employing a proper cooking and cooling environment by using thermometers.
- Microwave, cooked food appropriately.
- Proper refrigeration of cooked food within two hours of cooking, at 40 F.
- Keep cooked food at temp >140F.

FAST FACTS

Outbreak: Origin: unknown - "gas gangrene"
Mortality rate: low
Mode of transmission: spores, contact, GI tract, blood
Host: environment, soil and marine sediment
Symptoms: myonecrosis (necrotizing soft tissue infection)
Complications: life threatening muscle infection, anaerobic cellulitis

ENTEROHEMORRHAGIC FEVER
Hemolytic Uremic Syndrome-HUS 0157:H7 aka Hamburger's Disease

Definition:
HUS is an acute infection caused by eating uncooked-undercooked meat or drinking unpasteurized juices-drinks. *Escherichia coli* is a gram-negative, rod-shaped bacteria belonging to the genus Escherichia that commonly resides in the human colon. The strains of Escherichia Coli that cause ailments in humans are commonly known as enterohemorrhagic E. coli (EHEC). *EHEC serotype O157:H7* is a human pathogen found to be responsible for bloody diarrhea outbreaks and hemolytic uremic syndrome (HUS) worldwide.

Triad-Children
- Acute Kidney Injury
- Thrombocytopenia
- Hemolytic Anemia

Number of cases: 63,000 cases annually in the US.

Number of Deaths: 2,100 hospitalizations and deaths annually in the US.

Period:
Various outbreaks have been reported, usually during summertime, in association with county fairs where

hotdogs are popular food items especially amongst kids.

Etiology
It is caused by gram negative, rod-shaped bacteria, which belongs to *O157:H7* which is a gut commensal or flora. It is usually contracted by consumption of uncooked or undercooked hamburgers by Shiga Toxin-producing E Coli (STEC-HUS) or unpasteurized juices.

Epidemiology
90% of the acquired cases are caused by STEC-HUS, in children under age 5. There has been an unfortunate deadly outbreak in the US, which was related to unpasteurized apple juice.

Incubation Period
Typically, 3-5 days.

Transmission
Through contaminated meat products.

Clinical Manifestation
- Asymptomatic.
- Symptomatic.
    - Bloody diarrhea.
    - Abdominal pain.

Diagnosis
Clinical history-consumption of uncooked-undercooked meat or unpasteurized juices.

Treatment
- There is no specific treatment.
- Supportive treatment.
  - Water and electrolyte replacement.
- Blood product transfusions as needed.
- Plasma exchange.
- Dialysis
  - Hemodialysis.
  - Peritoneal dialysis (children).
- Bilateral nephrectomy
  - When associated with treatment-resistant malignant hypertension.

Prognosis
Favorable if early detection and intervention is employed.

Complications
- Renal complications are most pronounced if early intervention is nor delivered.
- Insulin dependent DM.
- Pancreatic insufficiency.

Prevention
- Good hygiene practices.
- Food safety assurance guidelines and programs.

FAST FACTS

Outbreak: Multiple associated with the county fairs and consumption of raw or
Undercooked meat "hamburgers", unpasteurized juices
Origin: unknown, but common in developed countries
Mortality rate: varies
Mode of transmission: food source - E Coli 01:H7
Host: humans - Humans
Symptoms: diarrhea, fluid and electrolyte imbalance, shock
Complications: hemorrhagic, the most common cause of renal failure in children

MARBURG VIRUS
aka Marburg "Germany" Disease

DEFINITION
It's a highly virulent, viral disease which is contracted by coming in direct contact with the infected bats or other carriers of the virus. It confers a very high mortality rate of around 83-90%.

Number of cases: 571 cases reported from 1967-2012.

Number of Deaths: Case fatality of 24-88% during various outbreaks. 470 deaths from 1967-2012.

Period: First recognized in 1967.

ETIOLOGY
Caused by a virus that belongs to the same family as that of *Ebola Virus*. The virus is contracted with prolonged exposure to caves inhabited by *Rousettus* bats, especially in spelunking enthusiasts. Once the virus is contracted, it can transmit from humans to humans via direct contact.

TRANSMISSIBILITY
- Blood, secretions, broken skin.
- Fomites, clothing contaminated with the infected secretions can also be the source of transmission.

Epidemiology
Two major outbreaks occurred in Marburg, Frankfurt in Germany and Belgrade in Serbia, former Yugoslavia, in 1967. It was supposedly caused by the green monkey *Cercopithecus aethiops,* which were imported from Uganda for the lab experiments. Later outbreaks were reported in Angola, Congo, Kenya and South Africa.

Incubation Period
2-21 days

Prevention
- Avoiding exposure to animals and African fruit bats that are known to be the carrier.
- Contact isolation to avoid human to human transmission.
- Barrier methods of isolation, gloves, gowns, masks and miscellaneous PPE.
- Isolate the PUI or infected person or animal- avoiding nosocomial spread.
- Proper sterilization of needles and other instruments, equipment.
- Avoiding spelunking in the endemic areas, i.e., Uganda.

Clinical Manifestation
Constitutional
- Fevers-sudden and high.
- Headaches.

CORONAVIRUS AKA COVID-19 - SARS-COV-2

- Malaise.
- Patient appearance has been reported as *"Ghost Like"*, sunken eyes, withdrawn and expressionless face, with extreme weakness and lethargy.

GI symptoms
- Abdominal cramps
- Nausea
- Vomiting
- Diarrhea (severe-watery)

Dermatological
- Maculo-papular skin rash on the torso.

Hemorrhagic diathesis
- Bleeding starts day 7 or later.
- GI sources, hematemesis or bloody diarrhea are the most common symptoms.
- Epistaxis
- Bleeding from gums or vagina may occur

Central Nervous System
- Confusion
- Irritability
- Aggressive behavior

DIFFERENTIAL DIAGNOSIS
- Typhoid.
- Malaria.
- Ebola (hemorrhagic manifestation mimic).

Diagnosis
- ELISA.
- Antigen testing.
- PCR-RT.
- Viral isolation by cell culture.
- Serum neutralization tests.
- IgM (recent-current infection), IgG (past-remote infection).

Treatment
- There is no specific treatment.
- Supportive
  - Supplemental oxygen.
  - Ventilatory support.
  - Fluid resuscitation oral or IV route.
  - Electrolyte replacement.
  - Bleeding control.
  - Transfusion of blood products or factors.

FAST FACTS

Outbreak: Multiple Germany, Serbia, Africa
Origin: unknown
Mortality rate: Few cases but highly virulent
Mode of transmission: virus shedding from the infected secretions
Host: humans - Humans - bats - primates
Symptoms: bleeding "Ghost Like Appearance"
Complications: hemorrhagic manifestations

CHOLERA
aka "water rice diarrhea"

DEFINITION
It is an acute infectious, diarrheal illness which is caused by *Vibrio cholerae*.

Number of cases: <10 cases are reported each in the US, as compared with the rest of the world which reports about 4 million cases.

Number of Deaths: 21,000 - 143,000 deaths annually worldwide.

Period: First pandemic occurred in 1817. There have been multiple outbreaks across the globe since the first outbreak.

ETIOLOGY
Caused by a gram-negative bacterium *Vibrio cholerae*.

EPIDEMIOLOGY
Cholera was prevalent in the USA in the 1800's. After the advent of modern water sanitation, sewage and treatment, it has practically been eradicated. Most common outbreaks in the US are caused by improperly handled and kept seafood. Cholera is prevalent in Asia, African and Latin America. Cholera outbreak in Naples, Italy led to practices of deep-frying food

like pizza, which is still prevalent in parts and streets of Naples.

INCUBATION PERIOD
Ranges from 2 hours to 5 days.

MODE OF TRANSMISSION
- Contaminated water and food sources are the primary mode of transmission in most of the world.
- Seafood, especially when obtained from the coral reef-in, is the major source in the USA, especially on the Gulf Coast.

MORTALITY
It is often fatal, if not treated earlier, promptly and aggressively, due to severe dehydration and electrolyte disturbances that ensue at the outset of the disease.

CLINICAL MANIFESTATION
- Explosive diarrhea, aka *"rice water diarrhea."*
- Vomiting.
- Extreme Thirst.
- Decreased urine output due to dehydration.
- Dehydration-up to 20 liters of fluid loss or deficit has been reported.
- Hypovolemic shock.
- Acute kidney failure.
- Septic shock.

- Muscle cramps.
- Seizures due to severe electrolyte abnormalities.

DIAGNOSIS
- Rapid Test
  - Crystal VC dipstick-filed test.
  - Stool sample for culture, as there are false negative dipstick tests.

CULTURE
- Stool test on TCBS (Thiosulfate-Citrate-Bile-Salts)-available in 24 hours.

TREATMENT
Supportive treatment
- More than 80% of patients will resolve with supportive management.
- Rehydration with Oral Rehydration Salts (ORS) or IV fluids approximately one liter per hour may be needed initially.
- Electrolyte replacement.
- Zinc sulphate.
- Homemade rehydration drinks.
  - One liter of boiled, or chemically treated water.
  - Half teaspoon of salt.
  - Six level sugar spoons.

Definitive Treatment
- Antibiotics
  - Doxycycline.
  - Azithromycin, erythromycin.
  - Tetracycline.
- Antibiotics are helpful in 20% of severe cases.
- Justified and timely use of antibiotics may reduce the duration of symptom and infectivity.

Prevention
Use of purified water is recommended, which is either boiled, chemically treated, or bottled.

This water is used for:
- Drinking.
- Food preparation or drinks.
- Ice making.
- Brushing teeth, washing face and hands.
- Dish washing.
- Washing fruits and vegetables and other edibles.

How to disinfect water:

Boil it for one minute to three minutes depending on the altitude or filter it and use a commercial chemical disinfectant. Avoid raw foods, including the following:
- Unpeeled vegetables and vegetables.
- Unpasteurized milk and milk products.
- Raw or undercooked meat or shellfish.

- Fish caught in tropical reefs, which may be contaminated with vibrio.

VACCINATION

Adult vaccines are available and recommended, when travelling to high-risk endemic areas.

FAST FACTS
Outbreak: Multiple in the underdeveloped countries - Haiti 2010
Origin: unknown - more common in the underdeveloped countries
Mortality rate: 100,000 - >3 million cases a year
Mode of transmission: fecal-oral route
Host: humans - Humans
Symptoms: diarrhea, fluid and electrolyte imbalance, shock
Complications: hypovolemic shock

Legionnaires Disease
aka Legionella "Air Conditioner Disease"

DEFINITION
An acute respiratory illness caused by atypical respiratory bacteria, spread by bacteria which is carried in the infected water sources, especially in the form of a mist.

Number of cases: 70,000 annually with about 18,000 hospitalizations.

Number of Deaths: 10% mortality-varies from year to year.

PERIOD:
- 1976-Philadelphia-USA 221 cases with 34 deaths.
- 2003-Pes De Calais-France 86 cases with 18 deaths.

ETIOLOGY
Caused by gram-negative bacteria with *L Pneumophila*. It is common in soil and aquatic environments. There are about 50 species with multiple subtypes.

INCUBATION PERIOD
Days to weeks.

Mode of Transmission
It is spread by contaminated water sources, I.e., air conditioners, swimming pools, ice making machines, windshield washer fluid or fountains. There is no person-to-person spread of the disease. The spread of disease is usually airborne and can travel up to 6 miles from the contaminated source once airborne.

History
Legionnaire's Disease was first recognized when a group of veterans in a hotel presented with similar respiratory illness with some with pneumonia. It was a conference of American Legions, hence the name "Legionnaires Disease". About 221 attendees staying at the same hotel in Philadelphia in 1976 got infected and 34 died.

Clinical Manifestation
- Cough.
- Fever "Pontiac Fever."
- Gastrointestinal symptoms, abdominal pain, diarrhea.
- Shortness of breath.
- Respiratory distress or failure.

Diagnosis
- Constellation of clinical symptoms.
- Urinary or serum legionella antigen.

Treatment
- Azithromycin.
- Fluoroquinolones i.e., Levaquin or Moxifloxacin (preferred agent in patients with co-morbid conditions or disease burden).

Mortality
Associated with complications of pneumonia or respiratory failure, especially in patients with underlying lung conditions i.e., COPD or immunocompromised status cancer or chemotherapy.

Vaccines
There is no vaccine available.

Control Measures
- Chemical.
- Thermal
    >50 degree Celsius.
    <25 degree Celsius.
  UV Light Sources.

Bio-terrorism
Legionella can be genetically modified to enhance its lethality to 100%.

CORONAVIRUS AKA COVID-19 - SARS-COV-2

FAST FACTS
Outbreak:
Origin: developed countries
Mortality rate: 10% - 70,000 cases per year
Mode of transmission: contaminated water source - Air Conditioners
Host: environment
Symptoms: respiratory symptoms
Complications: respiratory failure, pneumonia

PRION DISEASES
Creutzfeldt-Jakob Disease (CJD) aka "Mad Cow Disease"
"Kuru" aka cannibalism

Fatal Familial Insomnia (FFI)
Gerstmann-Straussler-Scheinker Syndrome (GSS)

DEFINITION
These are fatal, rapidly progressive neurocognitive and neurodegenerative diseases caused by a protein moiety called prion which cannot be classified as either bacteria or a virus. These diseases often have prolonged half-lives.

Number of cases: 1.5 cases per million per year.

Number of Deaths: almost fatal within two years.

Period: 1996 was a major outbreak in the UK. Kuru was reported many years ago, in association with the tribal custom of consumption of the brain of their ancestors, in Papua New Guinea.

INCUBATION PERIOD
It is in the years both in cows and humans. There have been reports of manifestation of the disease 50 years after its infliction.

Mode of Transmission
- Inherited.
- Consuming contaminated meat "Implicated in the Mad Cow Disease."
- Organ transplantation.
- It is not contagious as from humans to humans.

Mortality
Nearly 100% by 1 year after getting infected and the disease onset.

Classification
Classic Type (CJD)
- Conventional disease is 10-15 percent.
- Elderly 60-70's are more commonly affected.
- Short illness duration 4-5 months.

Variant Type (vCJD)
- Also known as *Bovine Spongiform Encephalopathy (SPE)*, often called mad cow disease. The first outbreak was reported in 1996 in the United Kingdom.
- Younger people in the 20's are commonly affected.
- Prolonged illness duration year or longer.
- Peculiar MRI findings on thalamus, T2, diffusion weighted images.

Iatrogenic Type
- Brain surgery instrumentation.
- Dura mater and corneal growth.
- Contaminated human growth hormone.
- Since 1979, there have been no more cases reported due to strict autoclave techniques.

Familial Type
- Hereditary transmission.

CLINICAL MANIFESTATION
Neurological issues including:

Early Symptoms
- Memory
- Behavior
- Coordination
- Speech

Late Symptoms
- Visual disturbances.
- Dementia.
- Involuntary movement disorder.
- Coma.

PSYCHIATRIC-PSYCHOLOGICAL MANIFESTATIONS
- Anxiety
- Depression

Diagnosis
- CSF (Cerebrospinal Fluid).
- Western Blot Protease Resistant PrP.
- EEG (Electroencephalogram).
- MRI.
- Brain biopsy.

Cause of Death
- Respiratory failure
- Heart failure
- Pneumonia

Treatment
- There is no specific treatment.
- Supportive care, including oxygen, hydration and infection control, prevention and treatment remains the mainstay treatment modalities.

Kuru
This disease was endemic in certain tribes (Fore) in Papua New Guinea. The transmission was from person to person, in conjunction with the cannibalistic rituals of eating ancestral remains or the brain. This practice has vastly disappeared after the ritual practices abated in the 1950s. However, there have been some reports of disease as late as in the 1990's which could be attributed to a prolonged incubation period of more than 50 years, after cessation of human cannibalism

practices in Papua New Guinea. Hallmark of the disease is progressive neurological decline to a total incapacitation. Death ensues as a result of inability to move, bedridden status and respiratory complications i.e., pneumonia.

Gerstmann-Straussler-Scheinker Syndrome (GSS)

This is another familial neurodegenerative prion disease, which has an autosomal dominant pattern of transmission. It predominantly affects the cerebellum and results in an array of neurological manifestations including ataxia, gait disturbances. As the disease advances, it affects the cognitive areas of the brain resulting in dementia and progressive leg weakness. Death follows within five years of neurological symptom onset. The diagnosis relies on demonstration and identification of the PRNP mutations.

Familial Fatal Insomnia

This is an autosomal dominant disease hereditary condition which is present in sporadic families. This is progress disease which presents with insomnia and loss of normal circadian pattern of sleep. It leads to progressive neurological decline and dementia. This is an ultimately fatal disease. Diagnosis is usually by genetic testing. There is no treatment available.

FAST FACTS

Outbreak: small cluster of diseases in kindreds - "mad cow disease" outbreak in
England 1996
Origin: developed countries
Mortality rate: low - long incubation period - years
Mode of transmission: contaminated meat, human brain in "kuru"
Host: humans, livestock "kuru" caused by practice of ritual cannibalism in
Papua New Guinea
Symptoms: dementia, neuropsychiatric manifestation, ataxia
Complications: progressive neurodegenerative disease - almost fatal condition

TRYPANOSOMIASIS
aka "African Sleeping Sickness"

Definition:
This disease got its notoriety from manifestation of unique symptoms which cause excessive daytime sleepiness.

Number of cases: 2000 cases reported in 2017-18, decreasing rapidly in current years.

Number of Deaths: 50,000-500,000 a year.

Period: first recognized in 1970.

Pathogenesis:
These are the protozoan hemoflagellates of the genus *Trypanosoma*, in the subgenus *Trypanozoon*.

Epidemiology:
There are two geographical locations, where this disease is endemic. Africa and South America.

Host:
Cattle, livestock i.e. goats, pigs and dogs are the primary host.

Transmission: Transmitted by bite of an infected *Tsetse* Fly - (pronounced 'see see fly").

- Glossina Species
  - Both male and female of the fly can transmit infection.
  - There are reports of maternal-fetal transmission.
  - Transmission, through sexual route, blood transfusion and organ transplantation also has been reported.
  - Bite usually occurs during the daytime.
  - Hunters and cattle herding are a risk factor for the local populace.
  - Safari tourists, Travelers and people visiting game parks are particularly at high risk.
  - This disease cannot be contracted outside the endemic areas, therefore if this disease occurs outside of these areas, a detailed travel history should be obtained.

Geographic Distribution:
- Predominant in the rural areas, savannah, forests and thick vegetation.
- Congo, Uganda and Sudan.

African Trypanosomiases
- East African Variety-More acute and aggressive
  - *Trypanosoma brucei rhodesiense*
- West African-Slow onset and chronic disease
  - *Trypanosoma brucei gambiense*

South American Trypanosomiasis (Chagas Disease)

INCUBATION PERIOD:
Days to weeks in the East African variety and years in the West African variety.

SIGNS AND SYMPTOMS:
A two stage disease:
 Stage- I *(Hemolytic Stage)*
- Painful, erythematous, skin rash which is oftentimes called *chancre*.
- Hematogenous and lymphatic spread.
- Development of constitutional symptoms, fever, malaise.
- Lymphadenopathy.

Stage-II *(Meningoencephalitis stage)*
Systemic spread -Central Nervous System.
- Mental:
    - Confusion, personality changes, delirium, anxiety, hallucinations.
    - Reversal of nocturnal circadian rhythm to excessive daytime sleepiness.
    - Seizures and coma.
- Sensory:
    - Anesthesia
    - Paresthesia
    - Hyperesthesia
    - Pruritus
- Motor:
    - Weakness

- Gait abnormalities
- Speech abnormalities
- Endocrine Abnormalities:
  - Hypothyroidism
  - Hypogonadism
  - Adrenal insufficiency
- Cardiac Abnormalities:
  - Myocarditis

Diagnosis:
- Presence of parasite
- Biopsy of the skin lesion or chancre
- Serologic and microbiological testing
- CSF analysis or a spinal tap
  - Diagnostic
  - Surveillance (every six months in chronic illness to ascertain treatment
  - effectiveness.

Treatment:
- This disease is ultimately fatal, unless treated timely and appropriately.
- There are chances for re-infection so having a disease once doesn't confer immunity.
- Pentamidine is the drug of choice and FDA approved.
- There are other drugs and drug-combinations available which can be requested if there are Issues getting pentamidine or allergies to the drug.

- Patients need to be monitored for 2 years or longer after treatment is initiated. CSF or body fluid surveillance for the absence of the trypanosomes every six months to assess efficacy of the treatment and disease relapse.

PREVENTION:
- Wear neutral colored clothing.
- Long sleeved, medium-thick texture clothing, as the fly can bite through thin fabric.
- Avoid going to thickets or bushes.
- Check for the *tsetse* flies in the surroundings, especially the vehicle before boarding.
- Insect repellent has not been proven effective.
- Vector control-more reliable method of controlling the population of the *tsetse* fly.
- Controlling reservoirs is often difficult due to the variety of reservoirs implicated in the disease.

VACCINATION:
No vaccine or prophylactic medication available to prevent the disease.

FAST FACTS

Outbreak: 1976
Origin: Africa
Mortality rate: 50,000 - 500,000 per year
Mode of transmission: *TseTse* Fly bite carries the parasite
Host: cattle and livestock
Symptoms: daytime excessive sleepiness, neurological and cardiac symptoms
Complications: untreated cases are almost fatal

AMERICAN TRYPANOSOMIASIS
aka "Chagas Disease" or Kissing Bug Disease"

DEFINITION:
A tropical disease which can result in cardiac and neurologic manifestation when a patient is bitten by *T. Cruzi*. This parasitic disease got its name from the Brazilian doctor Carlos Chagas.

Number of cases: 7 million infected worldwide.

Number of Deaths: 12,000 annually-mostly- Due to cardiac arrhythmias.

Period: First discovered in 1909.

PATHOGENESIS:
This disease is caused by *trypanosoma Cruzi*-commonly known as *"T-Cruzi."*

EPIDEMIOLOGY:
This disease is endemic and common in South America. Amazon basin, Brazil and Mexico are amongst the other 21 countries, where Chagas disease is endemic.

HOST:
Direct transmission to humans via the *Triatomine* bug, which is a type of reduviid bug. This bug is a cone-nosed insect which is commonly referred to as the "Kissing

Bug" as it is nocturnal and bites around the mouth or eyes. This bug lives in the walls and cracks inside the home. They come out at night for a blood feeding frenzy on their lips and eyes. It defecates and urinates at the bite site and introduces the parasite into the skin from where it is transmitted to the blood and organs.

Transmission:
It is vector-borne transmission which occurs via feces and urine of the Triatomine bug, which carries T Cruzi. Common mode of transmission is:
- Oral (food-borne illness).
- Blood, transfusion, organ transplantation.
- Maternal-Fetal.
- Accidental (lab accident).

Clinical Manifestation
- These vary from asymptomatic to systemic disorders.

Signs and Symptoms
Phase I - Acute Phase
- Mostly asymptomatic.
- Skin lesion at the bite, unilateral eyelid swelling.
- Constitutional symptoms, fever, malaise.
- Systemic symptoms, chest pain, shortness of breath, swelling, abdominal symptoms.

PHASE II - Chronic Phase
- Cardiac - 30%
  - Arrhythmias.
  - Congestive heart failure (most common cause of death).
- Gastrointestinal - 10%
- Neurologic

PUBLIC HEALTH CONTROL MEASURE
- Vector control-CDC recommends not killing the bug rather putting it in a jar and bringing it to a lab for identification.
- Spraying around houses and surrounding areas with insecticides.
- Screening blood before transfusion.
- General house cleaning measures.
- Use of bed-nets.
- Screening the transplanted organs.
- Maternal screening and treatment during pregnancy.
- Infant screening and treatment.

TREATMENT:
- Similar to its African counterpart, this disease is ultimately fatal, unless treated timely and appropriately.
- *Benznidazole* and *nifurtimox*- 100% effective even given within a few days of initial manifestation or during the acute phase of the disease. Both drugs are equally effective.

- This regimen is not recommended in pregnancy, kidney or renal failure.
- Also relatively contraindicated in patients with underlying neurological diseases.
- Efficacy goes down significantly if treated later in the disease process and in elderly population.
- Treatment is also suggested when there is reactivation of the disease, especially when the patient becomes immune compromised.
- Treatment duration could be up to 2 months, depending on the disease response and side effect tolerance.

VACCINATION

No vaccine is currently available for Chagas disease.

FAST FACTS

Outbreak: 1909 - "Chagas's disease"
Origin: South America
Mortality rate: 10,000 per year - 7 million reported cases
Mode of transmission: *kissing Bug* bite carries the parasite
Host: cattle and livestock
Symptoms: daytime excessive sleepiness, neurological and cardiac symptoms
Complications: untreated cases are almost fatal

LYME DISEASE
aka "Lyme Borreliosis" aka "Deer Tick Disease"

DEFINITION:
It is the most common vector borne illness in the US. It is an infectious disease caused by *Borrelia* bacterium, through a tick bite. It was first discovered by Dr. Burgdorferi.

Number of cases: About 500,000 worldwide.

Number of Deaths: Very few cases of Lyme's disease result in direct mortality.

Period: First recognized in 1982.

PATHOGENESIS:
This disease is caused by the *Borrelia Burgdorferi* bacteria and transmitted through a tick bite. Occasionally a close species, Borrelia *Mayonii* can rarely cause this disease. The vector is a black legged tick.

EPIDEMIOLOGY:
Lyme disease got its notoriety and name from the disease's initial manifestation and recognition in Lyme, Connecticut. White Tail deer are often the intermediate hosts. Anecdotal review hypothesizes that Lyme disease existed in the forests of North America about 60,000 years ago.

CLINICAL PRESENTATION:
Lyme disease can cause illness in both humans and other animals including dogs. The earliest disease manifestation often goes unrecognized. At times, a "Bullseye" rash manifests on the skin especially on the extremities or torso. The rash may occur weeks after the tick bite and presents as erythema migrans.

Stages of the disease
- Early Localized (3-30 days)
  - Rash- "bulls-eye."
  - Fever.
  - Headache.
  - Swollen Lymph Nodes.

- Early Disseminated (>30 days)
  - Joint pain-arthritis-arthralgia.
  - Stiff neck.
  - Facial paralysis or palsy.
  - Dizziness.
  - Shortness of breath.
  - Neuropathies.
- Late Disseminated (months to years)
  - Cardiac manifestations i.e., heart block and arrhythmias.
  - Neurological symptoms.
  - Musculoskeletal sequelae, i.e., arthritis, muscle pain, weakness etc.

Diagnosis:
CDC recommends two step testing strategies:

- ELISA-first test.
- Western Blot: Second or confirmatory test only when the first test is positive or equivocal.

A blood sample is drawn and tested for antibodies. If the initial test is negative no further testing is recommended. However, if the initial test is positive or equivocal, a second test is often recommended from the same sample drawn for the initial testing. The Lyme test is positive only when the first step is positive or equivocal and the second step is also positive. Since it takes weeks to mount an antibody response, therefore if tested early in the course of illness the test may come back as negative, i.e., false negative. However, once antibodies are formed, they remain in the system for an extended lifetime, therefore antibody testing is not recommended for evidence of cure. A false positive test for Lyme disease may occur when there is infection caused by other tick-borne illnesses, i.e., *Rocky Mountain Spotted Fever* or other bacterial or viral illness. Occasionally there is false positivity in conjunction with immune-mediated or connective tissue diseases.

Treatment:
- Remove the tick or its body parts from the skin gently with tweezers.
- Wash the area with alcohol or soap and water.
- Avoid using folklore strategies i.e., crushing, burning the tick or let it remain on the skin till it detaches by itself.

Neurologic Manifestation or arthropathies
- Doxycycline - IV or oral for 2-3 weeks.
- Ceftriaxone - IV or oral for 2-3 weeks.

Cardiac Manifestation
- Doxycycline - IV or oral for 2-3 weeks.
- Ceftriaxone - IV or oral for 2-3 weeks.
- Amoxil - IV or oral for 2-3 weeks.
- Electrophysiologic or surgical intervention may be needed for heart block or arrhythmias.

Prevention
- Avoid wooded areas if possible.
- Treated or DEET impregnated clothing.
- Check and examine for ticks on gear, people and pets, i.e., dogs.
- Showering within a few hours after returning from a potentially tick infested area.

FAST FACTS

Outbreak: 1982
Origin: North America
Mortality rate: unknown - 50,000 cases worldwide
Mode of transmission: *Tick Bite* carries the parasite
Host: deer "white tail"
Symptoms: bullseye rash, neurological, joint and cardiac
Complications: heart block

Primary Amoebic Meningoencephalitis
aka Brain-Eating Amoeba aka PAM

DEFINITION:
This is an uncommon illness in the US. It is an infectious disease which is caused by an amoeba which is transmitted by getting exposed to warm stagnant fresh water, lakes, canals and ponds in the tropical or hot climates. *Balamuthia mandrillaris* has been identified in the tap water and soil.

INCIDENCE AND PREVALENCE:
200 infections-70 in the USA.

DEATHS-CASE FATALITY RATE:
100%

ETIOLOGY:
This disease is caused by a single cell amoeba *naegleria fowleri which is* the most common culprit organism which is more common in the freshwater source. *N fowleri* is not a true amoeba, rather it is shapeshifting ameboflagellate excavate, which belongs to the genus *naegleria* and phylum *perchlorozia*. This is another amoeba, Balamuthia *Mandrillaris* which is not only found in the water sources but also in the soil. First case was identified in zoo-kept mandrill monkeys at San Diego Zoo.

Geography:
More common in South and Central America. Southern half of the US also harbors some contaminated water sources. Effect of global warming may also create more habitats for growth and proliferation of these amoebic species.

Pathogenesis:
It usually is associated with swimming in the contaminated freshwater bodies, in the warm climatic regions, canals, rivers, ponds. The amoeba gains entry and access through the nose to the brain tissue, where it can cause widespread destruction of the brain tissue by digesting the brain cells. Another amoeba is *Balamuthia Mandrillaris* source of transmission may be contaminated water used for nasal rinse and sinus drainage i.e., Neti pot.

Host Factors:
- Immune makeup
- Environmental factors
- Genetics

Signs and symptoms:
Slow Growing: *balamuthia mandrillaris* weeks
Fast Growing: *naegleria fowleri* 1-10 days

- Headaches
- Nausea-Vomiting

- Skin rash
- Stroke
- Brain hemorrhage

DIAGNOSIS:
- Imaging
  - CT scan of the head
  - MRI of the brain
- CSF analysis
- Brain Biopsy

DIFFERENTIAL DIAGNOSIS:
- Challenging as present as upper respiratory viral infection
- Bacterial Meningitis
- Brain Tumor

TREATMENT:
- Ant amoebic therapy
  - Miltefosine
- Antibiotics
  - Azithromycin
  - Rifampin
- Antifungal
  - Amphotericin B

Often a fatal disease that progresses from mild headaches to catastrophic multi-organ failure. It usually is a *postmortem* diagnosis, as death ensues before a confident diagnosis is made and the treatment is initiated.

Prevention:

- Refraining from swimming in freshwater ponds, canals or rivers. Stagnant water seems to be more likely a source of amoeba, especially when watercolor is blackish and the bottom has loose sediment.
- Thoroughly clean medical equipment and instruments which are used with the water sources i.e., Neti pot, ENT apparatus, CPAP/BIPAP water reservoir or tubing.
- Avoid jumping into a warm water pond or lake, but if you pinch your nose or put a nose clip it may prevent splashing.

FAST FACTS

Outbreak: various cluster in the warm pools and hot water source
Origin: global
Mortality rate: almost fatal - few case "young population"
Mode of transmission: direct inoculation of the amoeba in the brain through upper airway or any break in the continuity of the skin "splash" in the contaminated Water source
Host: environment -water
Symptoms: neurological symptoms
Complications: untreated cases are almost fatal

LEISHMANIASIS
aka "Black Fever" aka Kala-Zar" aka "Dandfly Disease" aka "Neglected Tropical Disease-NTD"

DEFINITION:
Leishmaniasis is an infection caused by the *leishmania* parasite, which is transmitted by sandflies to its definite host Humans and dogs.

Number of cases: 700,000 to 1.2 million every year.

Number of Deaths: 20,000 to 30,000

EPIDEMIOLOGY:
Leishmaniasis is common in the tropics, subtropics often known as Neglected Tropical Disease" or NTD. Its habitat can range from rain forests to deserts. It is more prevalent in the rural areas than the urban locale. The disease has manifested in literally every continent except Australia and Antarctica. There have been cases reported in North America, but it is primarily related to travel to the high-risk areas in Central and South America, i.e., Costa Rica. The regions where it is endemic or has manifested over the years
- Southern Europe
- South America
- Southeast Asia
- Sub-Saharan Africa

- North Africa
- Middle east

Mode of Transmission: *Leishmania* parasite is carried by female *phlebotomine* sandflies and transmitted through the bite in both humans and dogs. There is no transmission from the dog to humans or vice versa. Also, it's not contagious so there is no human-to-human transmission. There are more than 20 species of *Leishmania* and its vector *phlebotomine*. *L donovani* is one of the most common species causing the disease.

Pathogenesis: Once the sandfly bite on the exposed skin surface, it creates an allergic reaction on the skin resulting in the release of histamine, which causes itchy rash, which can turn into a peculiar skin reaction papule, nodule or ulcers. Sandflies can also lay eggs on the skin.

Host:
- Humans
- Dogs and rodents

Classification:
- Cutaneous-superficial
  - Skin
  - Soft tissues
- Visceral-deep-*kala-zar*
  - Liver, spleen, bone marrow

Onset and Duration:
May take months or years to develop and manifest its disease. Skin lesions are the earliest manifestation.

Clinical Signs and Symptoms

Generalized Symptoms
- Fever - black fever
- Malaise

Cutaneous Leishmaniasis
- Lesions form at the bite site-usually exposed skin.
- Papules-nodules-ulcers with a crater which does not heal easily "volcano ulcer".

Mucosal Leishmaniasis
- Mouth and Nose.

Visceral Leishmaniasis
- Hepatosplenomegaly.

Diagnosis:
- Antibody Testing-serology.
- Molecular testing-skiing or visceral sample.
- Direct microscopy.

TREATMENT:

Cutaneous Leishmaniasis
- If it's self-limiting and confined, observation may suffice. Local skin and wound care may be all that's needed.
  - Pentamidine
  - Cryotherapy-Local Nitrogen treatment
  - Thermotherapy
  - Sodium Stibogluconate injection

Visceral Leishmaniasis
Individualized treatment approach is recommended as its success relies on the species, types of disease manifestation, and the host make up i.e., age, pregnancy and immune status.

Oral:
- Miltefosine
- Doxycycline
- Azoles- fluconazole, itraconazole

IV:
- Amphotericin B
- Paromomycin-aminoglycoside

PREVENTION & CONTROL:
- Full clothing-even thin layers can prevent a sandfly bite.
- Application of antibacterial oils or Dettol.

CORONAVIRUS AKA COVID-19 - SARS-COV-2

FAST FACTS

Outbreak: endemic in desert environment - Africa - Asia
Origin: Africa, Middle east
Mortality rate: 30,000 per year - 1.2 million cases
Mode of transmission: *Sandfly* Fly bite carries the parasite
Host: human - dogs
Symptoms: Volcano ulcer, skin rash, liver, spleen and bone marrow
Complications: *kala azar*

Abbreviations

Ag	Antigen
Ab	Antibody
ARDS	Acute Respiratory Distress Syndrome
Bac	Bacteria
Bc	Bacillus
PPE	Personal Protection Equipment
PAPR	Powered Air Purifying Respirator
H	Hemagglutinin
N	Neuraminidase
H1N1	Hemagglutinin-1, Neuraminidase-1 (Flu)
SARS	Severe Acute Respiratory Syndrome
SARS-CoV-2	Severe Acute Respiratory Syndrome Coronavirus type two
MERS	Middle Eastern Respiratory Syndrome
COVID-19	Coronavirus Disease of 2019
CSF	Cerebral Spinal Fluid
MRI	Magnetic Resonance Imaging
CXR	Chest X-Ray

ABBREVIATIONS

CT	Computed Tomography
PET	Positron Emission Tomography
CDC	Center for Disease Control
WHO	World Health Organization
EKG/ECG	Electrocardiogram-electrocardiography
GI	Gastrointestinal
CVS	Cardiovascular System
CNS	Central Nervous System
PNS	Peripheral Nervous System
Inj	Injection
PCR	Polymerase Chain Reaction
WB	Western Blot
ELISA	Enzyme Linked Immunoassay
TB	Tuberculosis
HAV	Hepatitis A Virus
HBV	Hepatitis B Virus
HCV	Hepatitis C Virus
HDV	Hepatitis D Virus
HEV	Hepatitis E Virus
CBC	Complete Blood Count
BMP	Basic Metabolic Panel
CMP	Complete Metabolic Panel
LFT	Liver Function Test
Bil	Bilirubin
TSH	Thyroid Stimulating Hormone
PCN	Penicillin
ACE-I	Angiotensin Converting Enzyme-Inhibitor
ARB	Angiotensin Receptor Blocker

ALI	Acute Lung Injury
VENT	Ventilator
TRALI	Transfusion Related Acute Lung Injury
TACO	Transfusion Associated Circulatory Overload
PUI	Patient or Person Under Investigation (suspected case)
EEG	Electroencephalogram
CSF	Cerebrospinal Fluid
MRI	Magnetic Resonance Imaging
CT	Computerized Tomography
PET	Positive Emission Tomography
NIPPV	Non-Invasive Positive Pressure Ventilation
BIPAP	Bilevel Positive Pressure Airway Pressure
CPAP	Continuous Positive Airway Pressure
AVAPS	Average Volume-Assured Pressure Support
PEEP	Positive End Expiratory Pressure
DEET	N-Diethyl-meta-toluamide or diethyltoluamide
MMR	Mortality and Morbidity Reviews
MMWR	Morbidity and Mortality Weekly Report (published by CDC)
FDA	Federal Drug Agency
DEA	Drug Enforcement Agency
OPV	Oral Polio Vaccine
ECMO	Extra Corporeal Membrane Oxygenation

ABBREVIATIONS

RNA	Ribonucleic Acid
DNA	Deoxyribonucleic Acid
ELISA	Enzyme Linked Immunoassay
PCR-RT	Polymerase Chase Reaction-Reverse Transcriptase
ORS	Oral Rehydration Salt
ICH	Intracranial Hemorrhage
SDH	Subdural Hematoma

References

THE COUNCIL OF STATE AND TERRITORIAL EPIDEMIOLOGIST(CSTE) CRITERIA FOR A PROBABLE COVID-19 CASE: https://wwwn.cdc.gov/nndss/conditions/coronavirus-disease-2019-covid-19/case-definition/2020/08/05/

Infectious Diseases Society of America Guidelines on the Diagnosis of COVID-19 https://www.idsociety.org/practice-guideline/covid-19-guideline-diagnostics/

American Academy of Otolaryngology –Head and Neck Surgery. Coronavirus Disease 2019: Resources, Anosmia, Hyposmia, and Dysgeusia Symptoms of Coronavirus Disease. Mar 2020.

American College of Physicians: COVID-19: An ACP Physician's Guide + Resources. 20 May 2020.

Johnson JD, Theurer WM. A stepwise approach to the interpretation of pulmonary function tests. *Am Fam Physician*. 2014;89(5):359-3

REFERENCES

Wright B M. A miniature Wright peak-flow meter. Br Med J 1978; 2 :1627.

Nunn AJ, Gregg I. New regression equations for predicting peak expiratory flow in adults. BMJ. 1989;298(6680):1068-1070. 8

Leiner GC, Abramowitz S, Small MJ, Stenby VB, Lewis WA. Expiratory Peak Flow Rate. Standard Values for Normal Subjects. Use as A Clinical Test of Ventilatory Function. Am Rev Respir Dis. 1963 Nov; 88:644–651.

Aeromedical Electronic Resource Office https://www.med.navy.mil/sites/nmotc/nami/arwg/pages/aeromedicalelectronicresourceoffice(aero).aspx

Manual of the Medical Department, NAVMED P-117, Chapter 15.

American College of Physicians: COVID-19: An ACP Physician's Guide + Resources. 20 May 2020.

UpToDate, Coronavirus disease 2019 (COVID-19): Clinical features:
https://www.uptodate.com/contents/coronavirus-disease-2019-covid-19-clinical-features

A Game Plan for the Resumption of Sport and Exercise After COVID-19 Infection. https://jamanetwork.com/journals/jamacardiology/fullarticle/2766124

QT Interval Measurement: Evaluation of Automatic QTc Measurement and New Simple Method to

Calculate and Interpret Corrected QT Interval Anesthesiology. 2006;104(2):255-260.

Patel PJ, Borovskiy Y, Killian A, et al. Optimal QT interval correction formula in sinus tachycardia for identifying cardiovascular and mortality risk: Findings from the Penn Atrial Fibrillation Free study. *Heart Rhythm*. 2016;13(2):527-535. doi: 10.1016/j.hrthm.2015.11.008

LA Times Airline pilots making in-flight errors-COVID-related Inaction

KTLA Pilots Making In-Flight Errors "Feeling Rusty"

Aronson, N., Herwaldt, B.,et al. Diagnosis and treatment of leishmaniasis: clinical practice guidelines by the Infectious Diseases Society of America (IDSA) and the American Society of Tropical Medicine and Hygiene (ASTMH) Clin Infect Dis 2016;63:e202-e264.

Two cases of visceral leishmaniasis in U.S. military personnel—Afghanistan, 2002–2004 (April 2, 2004 / 53(12);265-268)

Update: cutaneous leishmaniasis in U.S. military personnel—Southwest/Central Asia, 2002–2004 (April 2, 2004 / 53(12);264-265)

Cutaneous leishmaniasis in U.S. military personnel—Southwest/Central Asia, 2002–2003 (October 24, 2003 / 52(42);1009-1012)

REFERENCES

Unexplained illness among Persian Gulf War veterans in an Air National Guard Unit: preliminary report — August 1990-March 1995 (June 16, 1995 / 44(23);443-447)

Viscerotropic leishmaniasis in persons returning from Operation Desert Storm — 1990 – 1991 (February 28, 1992 / 41(08);131-134)

Jha AK, Duncan BW, Bates DW. Simulator based training and patient safety in: Making health care safer: a critical analysis of patient safety practices. *Agency for Health care, Research and Quality, US dept of Health and Human Services.* 2001:511–8. [Google Scholar]

Gaba D. Human work environment and simulators. In: Miller RD, editor. *In Anaesthesia.* 5th Edition. Churchill Livingstone: 1999. pp. 18–26. [Google Scholar]

Gaba D. The future of simulation in health care. *Qual Saf Health Care.* 2004;13:2–10. [PMC free article] [PubMed] [Google Scholar]

Lateef F. What's new in emergencies, trauma, and shock? Role of simulation and ultrasound in acute care. *J Emerg Trauma Shock .* 2008;1:3–5. [PMC free article] [PubMed] [Google Scholar]

Shapiro MJ, Morey JC, Small SD, Langford V, Kaylor CJ, Jagminas L, et al. Simulation based teamwork training for emergency department staff: does it improve clinical team performance when added to an existing didactic teamwork curriculum? *Qual Saf Health Care.* 2004;13:417–21. [PMC free article] [PubMed] [Google Scholar]

International Journal of Infectious Disease

The Next Pandemic-Ali S Khan

Epidemics and Society-Frank Snowden

CDC-Center for Disease Control

NIH-National Institute of Health

FDA-Food and Drug Administration

WHO-World Health Organization

MMWR-Morbidity and Mortality Weekly Review

UpToDate

Wikipedia

Mayo Clinic Review

BMJ-British Medical Journal

ACCP-American College of Chest Physician

Journal of Critical Care Medicine-JCCM

New England Journal of Medicine-NEJM

Journal of Society of Critical Care Medicine

Concise Review of Trauma, Critical Care and Emergency Medicine

Wall Street Journal

Apple News

REFERENCES

National Public radio-NPR

Fox News

Cable News Network-CNN

Washington Post

National Broadcasting Corporation-NBC

BBC Science Focus Magazine

Popular Science

Kaiser Health

Cleveland Clinic

Guardian

Sky News

The Atlantic

New York Times

Chicago Tribune

Time Magazine

National Geographic

International Policy Digest

Daily Mail

Newsweek

CBS

Business News

Peoples Magazine

American Journal of Transplantation Accepted Articles

Donor To Recipient Transmission Of SARS-CoV-2 By Lung Transplantation Despite Negative Donor Upper Respiratory Tract Testing D.R. Kaul A.L. Valesano J.G. Petrie R. Sagana D. Lyu J. Lin E. Stoneman

Characterization of hospital airborne SARS-CoV-2 Rebecca A. Stern, Petros Koutrakis, [...]Eric Garshick Respiratory Research volume 22, Article number: 73 (2021) Cite this article

End of Days by Sylvia Browne

**Multiple sources, media, books, articles were used as reference for the compilation of this review. Every effort was made to include and acknowledge the sources which were used as a reference. However, if sources and references are not mentioned in the acknowledgement section it is purely unintended and inattentional. Therefore, we ask for forgiveness due to lapse in our efforts to include everyone who was influential in putting this manuscript together. However, please reach out to the authors and publishers, if there was such a lapse and the reference was not mentioned, so we can make an effort to include that on the website and future editions and publications

Also by
Asif Anwar, MD

Concise Review of Critical Care, Trauma and Emergency Medicine

Concise yet up-to-date review of the most commonly encountered topics related to the critical care, trauma and emergency arena. All facets of medical profession may benefit, including doctors, nurses, pharmacists, respiratory therapist, physical, occupational, speech/language therapist. Emergency medical techs will also find it very useful in the field.

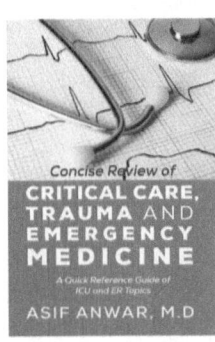

Fainting Pulse

Unlike other fields of medicine, with their occasional "oddities," the Intensive Care Unit sets the stage for a steady stream of unique medical challenges and patients who don't fit a standard profile. Fainting Pulse is a compelling compilation of stories based on these real-life cases—and told by the doctor who lived them.

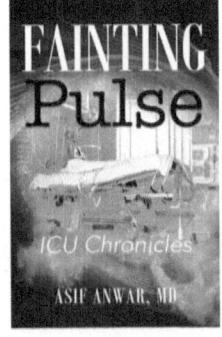

While some patients come and go from critical care quickly and uneventfully, others leave a permanent mark on their caregiver's souls. Among the dramatic stabbings, shootings, and freak car crashes, there are stories of exceptional patients and exceptional circumstances. Fainting Pulse shares some of these stories—from a woman struck by lightning to a man whose toothpick habit is nearly fatal; from swine flu to maggot therapy—with compassion, respect, and a healthy dose of humor.

LEARN MORE AT:

www.outskirtspress.com/concisereviewofcriticalcare
www.outskirtspress.com/faintingpulse

www.ingramcontent.com/pod-product-compliance
Lightning Source LLC
Chambersburg PA
CBHW031604210526
45464CB00004B/1426